Pest Control Technician
Safety Manual

Second Edition

Dedicated to the pest control technician, who never gets enough credit for being the heart and soul of the pest control industry.

Pest Control Technician
Safety Manual

Second Edition

Lawrence J. Pinto
Sandra K. Kraft

Pinto & Associates, Inc.
Mechanicsville, Maryland

Pest Control Technician Safety Manual

Title:	Pest Control Technician Safety Manual, 2nd Edition
Publisher:	Pinto & Associates, Inc.
	29839 Oak Road
	Mechanicsville, MD 20659-2201
	(301) 884-3020 (301) 884-4068 (fax)
E-mail:	Pinto_Associates@comcast.net
Web:	Techletter.com
Authors:	Lawrence J. Pinto, Sandra K. Kraft
Editor:	Sandra K. Kraft
Design:	Lawrence J. Pinto
Cover graphic:	© Gergana Todorchovska/iStockphoto

Copyright © 2006 by Pinto & Associates, Inc. All rights reserved. No part of the contents of this book may be reproduced or transmitted in any form and by any means without the express written permission of the publisher.

March 2000	First Edition
June 2000	Second Printing, First Edition
October 2006	Second Edition

ISBN 978-0-9788878-0-3

ISBN 0-9788878-0-8

DISCLAIMER

Please read the following statement carefully:

Pest Control Technician Safety Manual, 2nd Edition was published October 2006 by Pinto & Associates, Inc. Insofar as the information describes methods or procedures for pest control or safety practices, such information should be regarded only as suggestions or guidelines. The information is believed to be accurate as of the date of publication. The accuracy of the information, however, is not warranted by either the authors or Pinto & Associates. Each person using or distributing this publication is responsible for ensuring its accuracy and applicability at the time distributed and under the circumstances used or distributed. Further, the information contained in this manual is not intended to establish standards of care, nor is it intended to promote any single practice or procedure to the exclusion of others. No claim or warranty whatever is made or implied that the information, suggestions, recommendations, methods or procedures in this publication ensure safety, prevent injury, prevent property or environmental damage, or protect a company or individual from legal actions, lawsuits, or regulatory enforcement actions.

Deviation from the procedures described in this manual does not suggest that action has been improper under a given set of circumstances. There may be equally acceptable alternative procedures or methods to follow. Adherence to the suggestions or recommendations in this manual is not a substitute for careful review of safety hazards and procedures on a particular job, and compliance with federal, state and local requirements. The manual is merely intended to assist businesses and individuals in protecting their workers and themselves on the job. It is the responsibility of each individual, business, and organization to determine the appropriate methods or procedures to reduce hazards on the job, taking into account particular conditions at a job site, and applicable federal, state and local laws and regulations.

PREFACE

About seven million U.S. workers become injured or ill on the job each year. Each day, an average of 16 workers die from work-related injuries. Nearly all of these injuries, illnesses, and deaths could be prevented through training, safety programs, upgraded equipment maintenance, and proper supervision.

Pest control is not the most dangerous of jobs, but it's not the safest either. Some of the risks you face at work are obvious, often discussed at training sessions, in trade journals, and in company manuals. The best example is the wide range of hazards associated with using pesticides. Other risks are rarely considered, particularly those that are specific to certain types of pest control accounts. For example, do you service hospitals or nursing homes? If so, do you know how to protect yourself around communicable disease wards? From blood, bodily fluids, and needlesticks? From radiation and other biomedical hazards?

Do you take precautions when you work around asbestos pipe insulation? Do you know how to protect yourself from histoplasmosis in an old pigeon roost? Or hantavirus when controlling mice?

The risks faced by technicians are not necessarily extreme, but they are extremely varied, and in many cases depend on the types of accounts serviced.

The goal of any safety program is the prevention of accidents. Your first step in avoiding injury and illness on the job is to identify the hazards you face in your day-to-day work. Then, you either eliminate those hazards (often not possible in pest control when you work on someone else's property), control them, or avoid them. You control or avoid hazards by using protective equipment, such as respirators in enclosed treatment areas. You follow certain safety procedures, such as driving defensively, avoiding friable asbestos, using GFI's (ground fault interrupters) for electrical equipment in wet areas, and making it a policy never to reach under beds and furniture in hospitals and in drug-prone residences. Safety also means planning for emergencies, such as determining ahead of time what you would do in case of a pesticide spill.

The safest technicians mix knowledge with a good dose of common sense. Be alert to hazards, take proper precautions, wear the right protective equipment, ask questions, and keep safety in mind at all times. Finally, remember this rule: your personal safety is primarily your own responsibility.

Pest Control Technician Safety Manual

Contents

Preface vii
How to Use This Book xv
About Pinto & Associates xvi
    Techletter xvi
    Techletter.com xvi
    Consulting xvi
Accident Reporting 1
    Preparing an Accident Report 1
Alcohol And Drugs 2
    Alcohol and Legal Drugs 3
    Illegal Drugs 3
Allergy 6
    Insect and Mite Allergies 6
    Mouse Allergy 7
    Bird Allergy 8
    Allergy to Insect Stings 8
    Latex Allergy 10
    Peanut Allergy 11
Asbestos 12
    Common Sources of Asbestos 13
    How to Minimize Your Exposure to Asbestos 13
Attics And Crawlspaces 16
    Attics 16
    Crawlspaces 17
    Applying Pesticides in Attics and Crawlspaces 18

Bird and Bat Roosts 20
Bloodborne Pathogens 23
    Blood 24
    Bloodborne Pathogens and PPE 25
Compressed Gas Cylinders 27
    Precautions for Compressed Gas Fumigants 27
Confined Spaces 29
    What is a Permit-Required Confined Space? 29
    Whole Grain Storage and Processing 30
    Sewers, Storm Drains, Vaults 31
    OSHA Definitions Related to Confined Spaces 32
Driving and Vehicle Safety 33
    General Safe Driving Guidelines 33
    Special Rollover Precautions for Trucks and Vans 35
    Vehicle Accidents and Failing Eyes 37
    The "Two-Second Rule" 37
    Avoid Distractions 38
    Backing 39
    Requirements For DOT-Regulated Vehicles 40
    Inspection and Maintenance 41
    Jump-Starting 43
    Steer Clear of Static Electricity at Gas Pump 44
    Filling Gas Cans in Vehicles 45
    Pesticides in Vehicles 45
Electric Shock 49
    Grounded Equipment 49
    Ground Fault Interrupter 50
    Protecting Yourself When Drilling Slabs 52
    Connecting Plugs 53
    Contacting Electrical Circuits During Application ... 53

Pest Control Technician Safety Manual

    Aluminum Ladders 53
    Overhead Power Lines 53
    Industrial Sites. 55
    Working Outside in Thunderstorms...Just Don't. 55
Ergonomics and Musculoskeletal Disorders 57
    Risk of Musculoskeletal Disorders in Pest Control 58
    Hand-Arm Vibration Syndrome 59
Fiberglass Insulation 61
    Precautions When Working Around Insulation 61
Fire 63
    Fire Emergency Procedures 63
    Fires Involving Pesticides 64
    Fire Extinguishers. 64
    Pesticide Flash Point. 66
Firearms. 68
    Airguns 69
First Aid. 70
    Recommendations Related to CPR 71
    Recognizing a Heart Attack 71
Flashlights 73
    Heat from Halogen Bulbs 74
Hand and Power Tools 74
    Hand Tools 74
    Power Tools. 75
Head Injury 81
Heat and Cold 83
    Heat Illness 83
    Cold Weather Injuries. 84
Hookworm or "Creeping Eruption" 86
Hospitals And Other Medical Facilities 88

Ladders	89
Inspection	89
Ladder Placement	90
Precautions When Using Ladders	90
Step Ladders	91
How to Raise and Lower an Extension Ladder	91
Using Ladders Around Electricity	92
Lifting and Back Safety	93
Lockout/Tagout	95
Molds	96
Health Effects	97
Toxic Mold	97
Potential Mold Exposure for Pest Control Technicians	98
Personal Protection Against Mold	98
Natural Gas	99
If You Smell Natural Gas...	100
Gas Connectors on Appliances	101
Needlesticks	102
Noise	105
Reducing the Volume or Duration of the Noise	105
Pesticides And Other Chemicals	107
Hazard Communication Standard	107
MSDS	108
Toxicity	110
Applicator Risks by Formulation	112
Gasoline	113
PCBs	115
Pesticides and Terrorism	115

Pest Control Technician Safety Manual

Pesticide Poisoning 117
    Skin (Dermal) Exposure 118
    Oral Exposure 120
    Inhalation Exposure 122
    Eye Exposure 123
Pesticide PPE 125
    Choosing Protective Equipment 125
    Respirators 127
    Gloves 132
    Eye Protection 134
    Clothing 137
Pets and Guard Dogs 140
    Pets 140
    Guard Dogs 141
    Know What to Do When Confronted by a Dog 141
    Treatment of Bites and Scratches 142
Poison Ivy 143
Power-Dusting and Power-Spraying 145
    Equipment Inspection and Maintenance 145
    Precautions When Using Power Sprayers and Dusters 146
Radiation 148
    Health Effects of Radiation Exposure 149
    Minimizing Radiation Exposure 149
Rodents 151
    Rodent Bites and Scratches 152
    Ectoparasites 152
    Rodent Allergy 153
    Rodent-borne Diseases 153
    Guidelines for Handling Rodents 156
    Guidelines for Cleaning Up Rodent-Infested Sites 157

Roofs	158
Scaffolds	161
Scaffold Standards	161
Slips, Trips, and Falls	163
Minimizing Injury During a Fall	164
Falls and Aging	165
Spills	165
Spill Management	166
Spill Assistance	169
Spill Control Kit	170
Damaged Pesticide Container	171
Replacing a Damaged Hose	172
Stinging and Venomous Pests	174
Bees and Wasps	174
Fire Ants	176
Stinging Caterpillars	177
Velvet Ants	178
Scorpions	179
Spiders	181
Snakes	182
Stress	185
Stress Management	186
Tetanus	188
Tick-transmitted Diseases	189
Lyme Disease	189
Rocky Mountain Spotted Fever	190
Ehrlichiosis	191
Tick Paralysis	192
Precautions in Tick Areas	192
How to Remove a Tick	193

Pest Control Technician Safety Manual

Tuberculosis (TB)	194
Vaccinations	196
Hepatitis B Vaccine	196
Influenza Vaccine	197
Lyme Disease Vaccine	197
Plague Vaccine	197
Rabies Vaccine	198
Tetanus Vaccine	198
Violence	199
Precautions Against Violence	200
Warehouses	201
Unsafe Activity on Docks	201
Forklifts, Hand Jacks, and Pallet Jacks	202
Improper Stacking of Products	202
Failure to Use Proper Personal Protective Equipment	203
Improper Lockout/Tagout Procedures	203
Unsafe Handling of Hazardous Materials	204
Warning Signs	204
Wildlife	207
Rabies	207
How Can You Tell if an Animal Is Rabid?	207
Bites and Scratches	210
Ectoparasites	211
Capturing Nuisance Animals with a Pole or Snare	212
Review Questions	214
Answers to Review Questions	244

HOW TO USE THIS BOOK

This book is both a technician's reference book and a safety training tool. It can be used as a self-help book by an individual, or as a textbook in a group training session. Each major section (headed all in caps: ASBESTOS, NEEDLESTICKS, etc.) is listed in alphabetical order and covers a safety issue that might be faced by a pest control technician. At the end of each section is a list of the key points from the discussion. At the back of the book are questions to help test what you have learned.

Each section reviews the major points about a particular safety issue and how to deal with it. It is impossible to cover everything about each topic in a book this size. If you need more information, use supplemental training materials, the Internet, special training sessions, and ask questions of your supervisors.

We had a number of options for organizing the material in this book. Generally speaking, industrial safety training manuals are grouped by hazard; most commonly, physical hazards, chemical hazards, biological hazards, and radiological hazards. Pest control safety training, in contrast, is typically organized as safety on the job, safety with pesticides, safe driving, safety with tools, etc. It also usually emphasizes safety as it relates to customers, the public, or the environment, not risks to technicians themselves. Neither method of organization seemed to fit the information in this book, especially given the way that technicians are trained "in-house" by most pest control companies. Both methods of organizing the material would also make it more difficult to use the book as a reference.

We decided to simply list the major sections in alphabetical order. They can then either stand alone, or be combined with others to organize a training session around related safety issues. For example, a half-day training session on power tools might combine the sections on hand and power tools, ergonomics and musculoskeletal disorders, electric shock, and noise. Or a training session on dealing with animals might include the sections on wildlife, pets and guard dogs, rodents, tick-transmitted diseases, and vaccinations.

If, after using this book for a while, you feel that some other method of organization would have been more useful to you, please contact us and tell us so. Also tell us if there are other safety topics you would like to see addressed in a future edition of this book. As always, we are most interested in the comments, suggestions, and criticisms of our readers.

ABOUT PINTO & ASSOCIATES

Pinto & Associates, Inc. has specialized in writing about the technical and business aspects of pest control since 1983. We publish various books and newsletters about pest control.

Techletter

Techletter® is a biweekly training letter for technicians. It's unbiased...free of advertiser influence. And it's brief, illustrated, easy to read and up-to-date. *Techletter* includes safety training features tied to OSHA and other regulations. Subscribers also receive...at no additional cost...the *Quarterly Review*, two pages of questions covering *Techletter* topics from the previous three months. *Techletter* is the heart of in-house training programs for pest control companies around the country... it's that complete!.

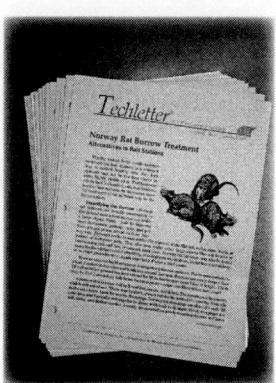

Techletter is the heart of in-house training for many companies

Techletter.com

Techletter.com is the website of Pinto & Associates, Inc. The website provides information on pests, pest control, and IPM for both professionals and nonprofessionals. Check out the articles on the website for the latest in pest control technical and business information. These articles change regularly.

Consulting

We provide a wide range of entomology and pest control consulting services to business and government. Our clients have included federal and state agencies, business associations, manufacturers, schools, and businesses with specific pest problems (property management firms, hospitals, nursing homes, hotels, etc.).

For a summary of our consulting services, see sections below.

Pest Control Publications

We develop and produce books, newsletters, training manuals, computer-based training, and videos for other businesses and organizations. Our work includes articles for magazines, company newsletter production, in-house training letters for pest control firms, manuals and books on pest control, computer-based training, and videos.

IPM Support

We actively promote IPM and provide IPM consulting, training and materials to industry, government, and other organizations.

Trouble-shooting Pest Problems

We provide trouble-shooting on difficult pest problems, technical specifications for pest control services, pest control oversight on large projects, and review of existing programs. Examples include rodents on large construction sites, bed bugs in multi-family housing, and flies in hospitals.

Pest Identification

We will identify a specimen of an insect or other arthropod for a fee. Our identification service is limited to urban pests in and around buildings (such as cockroaches, ants, flies, mosquitoes, stored product pests and other food pests, fleas, ticks, bed bugs, stinging insects, fabric pests, termites, and other wood destroying insects).

Field Research

Each year we do a limited amount of field research related to pest control. We follow Good Laboratory Practice Standards (GLPS).

Talks & Training Presentations

Larry Pinto is available for talks on a wide range of technical topics for pest control training sessions and other meetings.

For more information about our consulting services and publications, please visit our website at Techletter.com.

Pest Control Technician Safety Manual

ACCIDENT REPORTING

When an accident occurs, it's important to document the details, especially if there has been an injury or other impact on health. The report must be in writing. It may be called an incident report or an accident report, and it must be accurate. It may become the basis for an insurance claim, or a report to state regulators. It could be important for follow-up medical care, or if legal action is threatened. A detailed report can protect you and your company from unfounded accusations later.

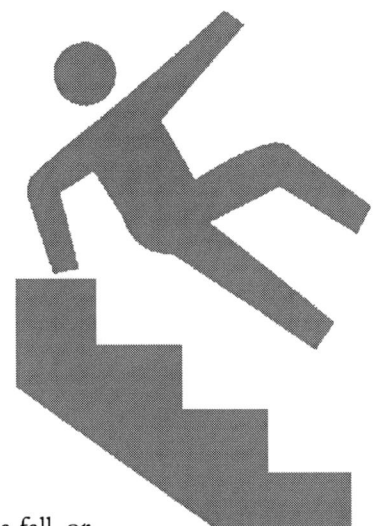

An accident may be a personal injury such as a fall, or accidental contact with contaminated blood while servicing a nursing home. It could also be a pesticide spill, or a fender-bender.

Preparing an Accident Report

Your company may have a standard form to use for this purpose. Some companies require that a supervisor fill out the official report. Regardless of who fills it out, it's important for you to note certain information about an accident before you forget details. Take care of any emergency situations first. Then, as soon as you get a chance, write down the following information:

Background information

Give details about the job or situation and the circumstances that led up to the accident. For example, this section answers the questions "who" (the names and affiliations of people involved), "where" (address of the customer or accident location), "why" (what was the job or visit for), and "when" (give exact time and date of the accident).

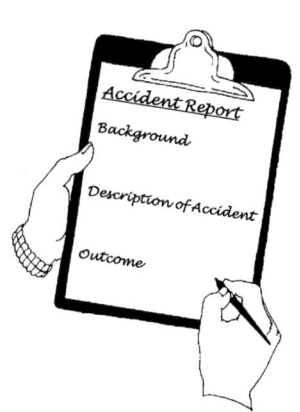

Description of accident

Provide details about what happened, in chronological order. Pretend that you're an unbiased eyewitness on the scene. Avoid giving personal opinion or speculations; stick to the facts. Describe any damage, illnesses, or injuries that occurred.

Outcome

Describe any actions taken after the accident. What was done to repair damage, clean up, tend to injuries, etc.? Give names and affiliations of any eyewitnesses, medical personnel, police officers, or others involved. List what still needs to be done to resolve the accident.

Finally, sign and date your accident report and give it to your supervisor at the earliest opportunity.

Key Points to Remember—Accident Reporting

- √ **Document the details of any accident resulting in an injury or health impact.**
- √ **Provide background information about the job and the circumstances that led up to the accident.**
- √ **Give details about what happened, in chronological order.**
- √ **Give names and affiliations of any eyewitnesses, medical personnel, police officers, or others involved.**

ALCOHOL AND DRUGS

Alcohol, illegal drugs, prescription drugs, and over-the-counter drugs can affect your ability to think, move, and react. Abusing them on the job can cause injuries, decrease productivity, and damage a company's image. Long term use of drugs and alcohol can have a cumulative effect on your body, sometimes permanent, that can alter job performance even if the substances are not actually used on the job.

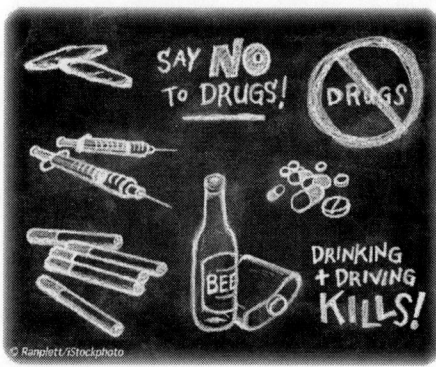

Photo © Ranplett/iStockphoto

Alcohol and drugs, when misused, can damage your health, hurt your family, and degrade your quality of life. If you must have a drink or a drug to get through life each day, you have a problem. Get help. Substance abuse assistance is available. Options include company programs (in some instances), your physician, alcoholism self-help groups, drug abuse rehab programs, or a health or addiction clinic.

Alcohol and Legal Drugs

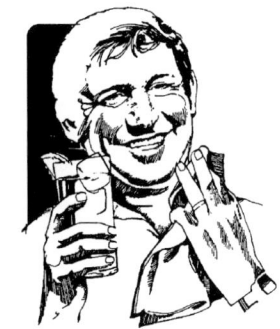

Alcohol is a drug. In fact, it's the drug most often abused by employees. It's as physically addictive as a barbiturate, as psychologically addictive as many tranquilizers, and as psychotoxic as LSD. It can affect your behavior, judgement, balance, blood pressure, cold perception, and coordination. Alcohol causes billions of dollars in damages, lost time, and lost lives from accidents and injuries on the job.

For certain types of work, even using a prescription or over-the-counter drug could cause significant risk to you, your coworkers, your customers, and the public.

Alcohol affects your judgement and balance

Antihistamines, for example, can cause drowsiness and loss of concentration and coordination. Tranquilizers may degrade job performance and reduce worker safety. Such drugs can make you more likely to injure yourself or others, more likely to take time off, and more likely to be operating below par. They can put you at risk when applying pesticides, using power equipment, working on a ladder, driving, or doing other tasks that require motor skills and judgement.

> *Check Your Company's Policy on Alcohol and Drugs*
>
> Your company probably has a policy about drinking alcohol on the job. It may also have a policy for over-the-counter and prescription drugs. Comply with those policies. If you need to take a prescription or over-the-counter drug that might affect your performance, be sure to inform your supervisor. You may need to be temporarily reassigned to other types of work.

Illegal Drugs

Illegal drugs...from pot to coke, from speed to ecstasy...create safety and health risks on the job. Drug users are slower to react to danger and are uncoordinated. They become forgetful and unable to judge time, space, and distance correctly. They make stupid errors, and have far more accidents and injuries. Illegal drugs are a major problem throughout the business world. Seventy-seven percent of drug abusers are gainfully employed, and 14 out of every 100 employees abuse drugs on the job. On average, twenty percent of employees between 18 and 25 years of age abuse drugs on the job.

> ### Consequences of Drug Use On-the-Job
>
> Drug users often claim they perform as well or better on drugs. Don't you believe it. Here are some hard statistics about workers who use illegal drugs:
>
> - They are $3^1/_2$ times more likely to injure themselves or another person in a work-related accident.
> - They are 5 times more likely to injure themselves off the job, in turn affecting performance or attendance on the job.
> - They are 5 times more likely to file a workers' compensation claim.
> - They are $2^1/_2$ times more likely to have absences of 8 days or more.
> - They are $^1/_3$ less productive.
> - They incur 300% higher medical costs.
> - About 50% of them engage in illegal activities.
> - About 25% of them steal from their employer.

Even a "casual" user of illegal drugs poses major health risks to himself and others. Furthermore, casual users often move to chronic drug abuse, moving from less serious drugs, such as marijuana, on to high-risk, highly-addictive drugs such as heroin or cocaine. Casual use all too often turns to addiction and desperation, stealing and dealing to support a destructive habit

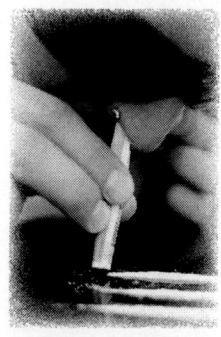

Drug users have far more accidents and injuries on the job

© Jean-Joseph Renucci/iStockphoto

Most companies have policies prohibiting their employees from using illegal drugs on the job and on company property, or whenever drug use impairs the ability to work or affects the company's reputation. Furthermore, by its very definition, illegal drug use is against the law. Many companies require that their employees take drug tests. Depending on company policy and state law, the tests might be given to all new employees, or be required after an accident, or be given randomly. Because of the dangers of drug use, and the impact of drugs on society, most workers now favor drug testing by their employers.

If a Coworker Has a Drug Problem

What should you do if you know a coworker has a drug problem? This is obviously a touchy situation. The Institute for a Drug-Free Workplace recommends the following actions:

> *What you should not do is look the other way. Drug abuse is naive (no one expects to become hooked), progressive, rooted in denial, and—as it progresses to severe stages—almost always fatal...*
>
> *You should not aid and abet drug users' progressive disease, make excuses for them ('it's temporary, he has problems at home, she's still a good worker, he can handle it, it's not as bad as it was'), or adopt their denial mentality.*
>
> *Be informed about the company's policy. Go to the coworker. Give them information, encouragement, understanding. Have them check it out, see what help they can get, and stand behind them. If need be, talking to his or her supervisor may save a drug abuser's life—and someone else's.*

— From *What Every Employee Should Know About Drug Abuse: Answers to 20 Good Questions.*
Published by the Institute for a Drug-Free Workplace

Key Points to Remember—Alcohol and Drugs

- √ **Alcohol and drugs affect your ability to think, move, and react.**
- √ **Alcohol is the drug most often abused by employees.**
- √ **Over-the-counter and prescription drugs can affect your safety on the job or when driving.**
- √ **Inform your supervisor if you take a prescription or over-the-counter drug that might affect your performance.**
- √ **Even a "casual" user of illegal drugs poses substantial health risks to himself and to others.**
- √ **Do not "look the other way" if you know a coworker has a drug problem.**

ALLERGY

An allergy is a high sensitivity to proteins and other substances in foods, plants, pollen, microorganisms, medicines, and insect parts. These substances are called *allergens*. An allergic reaction to such an allergen can be as mild as a runny nose or as extreme as death. Hay fever, for example, is a common allergic response to pollen. Anaphylactic shock is an often fatal reaction in cases of extreme allergy.

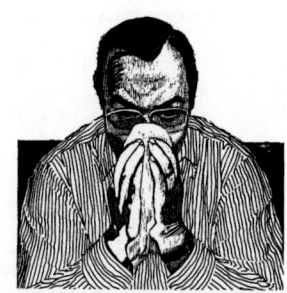
An allergy is the body's reaction to an "allergen"

Insect and Mite Allergies

Cockroaches, house dust mites, Asian lady beetles, fleas, and other insects and arthropods are known to produce allergens in their feces and body debris (cast skins, etc.). Other pests certainly do so as well. Repeated and prolonged exposure to these allergens can cause some people to experience mild hay fever-like symptoms of a runny nose and stuffed-up head, itchy dermatitis, or even stronger reactions leading to asthma.

Medical studies continue to show a steady increase in allergies and asthma among inner-city children who have been exposed to cockroach allergens.

Likewise, more and more people are reporting allergic sensitization to Asian lady beetles. In allergy skin prick tests, almost as many patients showed sensitivity to lady beetles as to cats or cockroaches. Sensitization to lady beetles was greater among patients living in rural areas compared to urban areas.

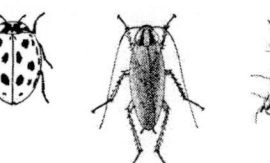

There have been no medical studies showing increases in pest-related allergies in pest control workers. Nevertheless, it makes sense to minimize your allergy risk. How? When doing intensive treatments ("cleanouts") of heavily infested accounts, or when otherwise disturbing large populations of cockroaches and other pests, wear a respirator and goggles and long sleeves.

Many insects and mites are known to trigger allergic reactions

Your respirator will filter out most allergens that may become airborne; it will filter all allergens if it is equipped with a *HE filter*. Long sleeves and long pants will help prevent contact dermatitis from insect parts.

Your goggles will keep the allergens out of your eyes. If you use a vacuum as part of your service, be sure it is also equipped with a HE or HEPA filter so that microscopic allergens do not become airborne.

> *HE Filter Versus HEPA Filter*
>
> An HE filter is a "high efficiency" filter...what used to be called a HEPA or "high efficiency particulate air" filter. HE filters are color coded magenta or red-purple—any N100, R100, or P100 filter is classified as an HE filter.

Mouse Allergy

Mouse allergies are far more common than once thought. Various studies in the past few years have demonstrated that mouse allergens (primarily mouse urinary protein), allergy to mice, and asthma associated with these allergies, are widespread, especially in urban inner-city areas.

For example, a study by the National Institute of Environmental Health Science (part of NIH), conducted in 75 locations across the United States, discovered the following:

- Mouse allergens exist in 82 percent of U.S. homes.
- Mouse allergens were found most often in the kitchen.
- High-rise apartments, mobile homes, and duplex-triplex residences had the highest concentration of mouse allergens.
- Mouse allergen presence increased with the age of the homes.
- Mouse allergen presence increased as household income decreased.
- Mouse allergen problems were not limited to urban, inner city areas.

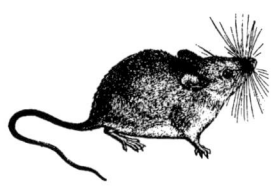

Mouse allergies are far more common than once thought

Another study, this by Johns Hopkins University conducted in urban inner-city areas, discovered that 95 percent of tested homes had mouse allergens in at least one room. The study found that 18 percent of the children living in these homes were allergic to mice and tended to have severe asthma.

Repeated and prolonged exposure to mouse allergens can cause those predisposed to allergies to experience hay fever-like symptoms of runny nose and stuffed-up head, itchy dermatitis, or asthma.

Given recent evidence about the high incidence of mouse allergies, technicians may need to take steps to protect themselves from mouse allergens. While there have been no studies showing increases in mouse allergies in pest control workers, it makes sense to minimize your risk of an allergic reaction.

> ### Precautions During Mouse "Clean-Outs"
> When doing intensive treatments ("clean-outs") of heavily infested accounts, using vacuums, moving furniture, or otherwise disturbing a mouse-infested area, technicians should wear a respirator equipped with an HE 100 level filter. It will filter out any allergens that become airborne. If your company uses vacuums as part of your service, they should be equipped with HE (or HEPA) 100-level filters to minimize airborne allergens.

Bird Allergy

There is a rare but dangerous allergy-related health threat associated with bird roosts. *Allergenic hypersensitivity pneumonitis* is a potentially disabling lung disease, not caused by an infectious agent, but by an allergic reaction to airborne debris from bird feathers, droppings, and other bird proteins. Experts estimate that from one to five percent of individuals exposed to bird proteins (antigens) will develop symptoms.

For safety information on working in bird roosts, see *Bird and Bat Roosts*.

Allergy to Insect Stings

Eight out of every thousand people suffer an allergic reaction to insect venom, mostly after being stung by a bee, fire ant, or wasp, such as a yellowjacket. Between 50 and 100 people die each year after having a severe allergic reaction to an insect sting. Just because you have never had such a reaction, does not mean that you never will, although the odds are against it.

> ### *"Normal" Sting Reaction*
> A normal reaction to a sting is not the same as an allergic reaction. The normal reaction is intense, immediate pain at the site of the sting, followed by localized swelling, warmth, and redness. These symptoms usually subside after a few hours but itching at the sting site may continue for days.

An allergy to an insect sting is serious. Sometimes an allergic reaction starts within minutes of exposure, peaks within 15-30 minutes, and is over within hours. The first symptom is a sensation of warmth followed by intense itching, often on the soles of your feet or the palms of your hands. Your skin flushes, hives may appear, your face swells, and it becomes hard to breathe. You may feel faint and anxious, with a sense of impending doom. Your blood pressure may drop. You are experiencing "anaphylactic shock," an acute, life-threatening allergic reaction. In some cases, people experiencing anaphylactic shock may have convulsions, become unconscious, and die.

Sometimes an allergic reaction to a sting is delayed, occurring hours or even a day after the sting. The reaction can include fever, hives, swelling at the site, headache, pain in the joints, and tender lymph nodes. This delayed reaction is usually less dangerous than an immediate reaction.

If you know or suspect you are allergic to insect stings, tell your supervisor. People who are highly allergic to insect stings are advised to avoid situations where they might encounter bees, wasps, and other stinging insects. Some carry special emergency kits, available by prescription, containing a premeasured epinephrine syringe or a special injector that automatically injects a dose when pressed against the thigh. Some kits also include a tourniquet and an antihistamine (to reduce allergy symptoms).

An allergic reaction may occur hours after the sting

> ### *Anaphylactic Shock Is a Medical Emergency!*
> If you think that you may be having an allergic reaction to an insect sting, see a physician. *If allergy symptoms appear immediately after you have been stung, it is a medical emergency. Get to a physician immediately or call 911.* Anaphylactic shock must be treated quickly, usually with an injection of epinephrine.

People who have had severe allergic reactions can sometimes be desensitized by injections of increasing amounts of the allergen over a period of years. A number of pest control workers have been successfully desensitized by this treatment, which is called "allergen immunotherapy."

See also *Stinging and Venomous Pests*.

Latex Allergy

Latex is natural rubber that is manufactured from a milky fluid from the rubber tree. A common <u>non</u>allergic reaction to latex safety equipment is the appearance of dry, itchy, irritated skin. In gloves, it is often the lubricant powder used inside the gloves that causes this reaction.

Some people have allergic reactions to the latex itself. For allergic people, symptoms usually appear within minutes of exposure. Allergic reactions can be mild (skin redness, itching, or hives), moderate (runny nose, sneezing, itchy eyes, scratchy throat), or severe (asthma or anaphylactic shock). Allergic reactions can be the result of direct skin contact, for example wearing latex gloves, or it can be the result of inhalation. When workers change gloves, the powder and attached protein particles can become airborne. The more a person is exposed to latex, the more likely he is to develop an allergic sensitivity. Note that several types of synthetic rubber may also be referred to as "latex," but it is only the natural rubber latex that causes allergic reactions.

> *Latex Allergy Precautions*
>
> To reduce your risk of developing a latex allergy:
>
> - Use gloves and products that are not made from natural rubber latex.
> - If you need to use latex gloves, choose powder-free gloves and look for gloves with a reduced protein content. "Hypoallergenic" latex gloves do not reduce the risk of latex allergy but they may reduce skin reactions to the chemical additives in latex.
> - When wearing latex gloves, don't use oil-based hand creams or lotions since they can deteriorate the gloves.
> - After removing latex gloves or other equipment, wash hands or face with a mild soap and dry thoroughly.
> - Clean any equipment or areas that may be contaminated with latex dust.

Although latex allergy is most common among workers in the health care industry, pest control technicians can be at risk from latex gloves. Latex gloves may be mandated when working in hospitals or similar sites for protection against infectious materials and other biohazards. Goggles and respirators may also contain latex.

If you think you've had a reaction to latex, notify your supervisor and see a physician.

Peanut Allergy

Why discuss peanut allergies in a pest control safety manual?

Because for many pest control technicians, peanut butter is a staple part of their service kit. It's useful as a food bait for many animals. It's smeared on snap traps or glue boards to catch mice and rats. It's mixed with rolled oats to lure larger animals like skunks and squirrels into traps. It's mixed with molasses as a bait for gophers and voles. It's even used as a food bait in some unusual ways to catch carp and other fish, deer, even starlings. Commercial toxic baits for rodents, ants, and some other pests use peanut butter or peanut meal as the food base. Basically, lots of animals like peanut butter and technicians like to use it because it's almost a universal bait.

Unfortunately, about 1.5 million people in the U.S. suffer from a severe allergy to the proteins found in peanuts. For a certain percentage of these people, even a minimal exposure to peanuts can result in life-threatening anaphylactic shock. Only about one in five people outgrow their peanut allergy over time.

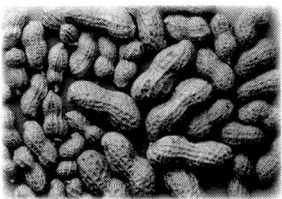

Many people are severely allergic to peanuts

Photo by ARS

Peanut allergy is a special problem for young children who may not be able to read food labels and may not understand which foods could contain peanuts, peanut oil, or peanut derivatives.

Cross-contamination is a particular problem in food plants. Many foods today are certified as peanut-free Do not use peanut-based baits when working inside food plants, since peanut residue could cause a cross-contamination.

Make it a habit to always ask your customer whether anyone, including pets, has allergies to particular foods or chemicals. If you do school IPM, make sure you ask the school nurse whether there are children present who have peanut allergies. If so, avoid the use of peanut butter or any commercial baits (including ant baits) that are peanut-based.

Also avoid peanut butter-based baits if any member of your family has a peanut allergy. You may carry back low-level peanut residues on your skin or clothes.

Key Points to Remember—Allergy

- √ **Certain people can experience an acute, life-threatening allergic reaction to an insect sting, food, or certain other allergens.**
- √ **If you think that you may be having an allergic reaction, get to a physician immediately or call 911.**
- √ **To reduce exposure to allergens from insects, mites, and mice when doing intensive treatments ("clean-outs") of heavily infested accounts, wear an HE 100 respirator, goggles, and long sleeves.**
- √ **Some people have allergic reactions to natural rubber latex in gloves, goggles, and respirators.**
- √ **If you know or suspect you are allergic to insect stings, latex, insect allergens, peanuts, or anything else in the workplace, tell your supervisor.**

ASBESTOS

Asbestos is a mineral fiber found in rocks. It has been used in many ways in construction and industry because it is fire-resistant, a good insulator, long-lasting, and not easily destroyed.

Some types of asbestos materials can break into small fibers that can float in the air. These fibers are so tiny that you cannot see them. Once inhaled, asbestos fibers can remain lodged in lung tissue for a long time. Over many years, these inhaled fibers increase the risk of lung cancer and other cancers, especially for smokers. There is a strong relationship between smoking and asbestos in causing lung cancer.

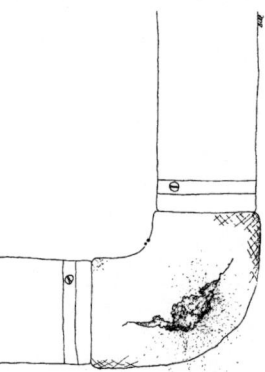

Breathing airborne fibers from crumbled, "friable" asbestos poses a cancer risk

In order to be a health risk, asbestos fibers must be released into the air. Soft, easily crumbled, friable asbestos poses the greatest risk. Asbestos that is undamaged is relatively safe, but it can become hazardous when sawed, sanded, drilled, etc. so that it breaks, crumbles, or disintegrates.

Common Sources of Asbestos

Asbestos was once commonly used in insulation and fire protection materials, so you may work around asbestos in older buildings. Common sources of asbestos include:

- Steam and hot-water pipe insulation (white cardboard-looking tubes; may be covered with cloth), and hot-air duct insulation (in a very thin layer)
- Wrapping around old boilers, coal/wood stoves, and furnaces (looks like plaster)

    Note: To be safe, presume that any thermal system insulation and surfacing material found in buildings constructed before 1981 contains asbestos.

- Wall and ceiling insulation (in some buildings built between 1930 and 1950)
- Attic vermiculite insulation made before 1990 and produced using vermiculite ore may contain asbestos fibers.
- Cement sheets, millboard, and paper on floor and walls around wood stoves
- Some acoustic ceiling tiles
- Vinyl floor tiles/sheet flooring manufactured before 1981 (always presumed to contain asbestos)
- Certain patching compounds and textured paints manufactured before 1977
- Ceiling coatings (mostly in apartments built or remodeled between 1945 and 1978)
- Roofing, shingles, and siding (asbestos siding looks like a rigid piece of corduroy)

How to Minimize Your Exposure to Asbestos

Whenever asbestos might be present in your workplace, take steps to minimize your potential exposure, particularly to asbestos fibers. Following are some guidelines when working around specific sources of asbestos.

Pest Control Technician Safety Manual

Asbestos Insulation Around Pipes, Boilers, and Furnaces

If the asbestos material is undamaged, no special safety equipment or precautions are necessary. Just be careful not to disturb or damage the insulation.

If the asbestos appears friable (soft and crumbling), notify your supervisor. Do not work in the area unless (1) you understand the risks you are taking and (2) you have been trained in proper safety procedures. Also, do not enter an area posted with a "DANGER ASBESTOS" sign without such awareness and training.

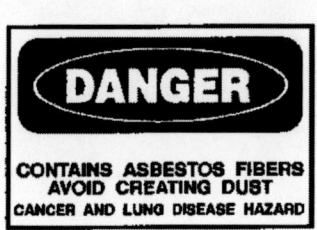

Do not enter a "Danger Asbestos" area without protection and training

Depending on the extent of the potential exposure, safety procedures in asbestos hazard areas are likely to include (1) wearing at least a half-mask, air-purifying respirator equipped with HE filters (color-coded magenta or red-purple—any N100, R100, or P100 filter is classified as an HE filter), (2) wearing protective clothing such as coveralls, gloves, booties, and hats, (3) special laundering procedures, and (4) using "decontamination areas" for disrobing and showering.

Drilling or Cutting Through Asbestos Floor Tiles or Sheet Flooring

In termite work, technicians often go through floor tiles and sheet flooring before drilling slabs. Presume that all vinyl floor tiles and sheet flooring contain asbestos if installed before 1981.

The best methods to access the slab through this material, with minimum exposure to asbestos, are to:

(1) If possible, lift tiles intact using heat (such as a heat gun).
(2) If not lifting an entire tile, cut off a corner or a plug while wetting the plug cutter, knife, or snip point.
(3) For sheet flooring, also be sure to wet the plug cutter, knife, or snip point when removing a section before drilling.
(4) If drilling through tiles or sheet flooring that might produce dust, use water sprays/mists to

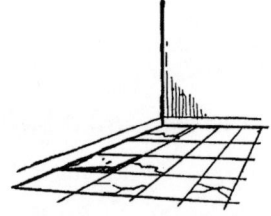

Presume that all pre-1981 vinyl floor tiles and sheet flooring contain asbestos

| 14 |

trap the dust. If there is any risk that the dust may become airborne, wear a respirator with an HE filter.

(5) Remove any excess dust by wet mopping or with a vacuum equipped with an HE filter.

Other Potential Asbestos-containing Material

Older buildings often have asbestos in wall and ceiling insulation, ceiling coatings, patching compounds, and textured paints. It is safest to assume asbestos is present and act accordingly. Use wet cutting and mists to keep down dust, wear a respirator if dust is produced, and vacuum up dust with an HE filter-equipped vacuum. If you suspect asbestos insulation is in an attic (some buildings built between 1930 and 1950), or a building with vermiculite insulation in the attic, do not power-dust the attic or disturb the insulation.

Key Points to Remember — Asbestos

- √ **Asbestos was once used in insulation, for fire protection, and in some flooring, ceilings, paints, and siding.**
- √ **Asbestos fibers inhaled into lungs increase the risk of lung cancer, especially for smokers.**
- √ **Soft, easily crumbled ("friable") asbestos material poses the greatest risk, while asbestos that is undamaged is relatively safe.**
- √ **Undamaged asbestos-containing material can become hazardous when sawed, sanded, drilled, etc. so that it breaks, crumbles, or disintegrates.**
- √ **Do not enter or work in an area with friable asbestos unless (1) you understand the risks you are taking and (2) you have been trained in proper safety procedures.**
- √ **In termite work, presume that all vinyl floor tiles and sheet flooring contains asbestos if they were installed before 1981.**
- √ **When in doubt, assume asbestos is present and act accordingly.**
- √ **When disturbing asbestos, wear an HE respirator.**
- √ **Do not power-dust an attic with vermiculite insulation or where you suspect other asbestos-containing insulation.**

ATTICS AND CRAWLSPACES

Pest control service commonly includes inspection or service in attics and crawlspaces. Technicians face numerous safety hazards in both locations. Some of those hazards are obvious, and some are not.

Attics

Ladders leading to attics are frequently broken, weakened, and dangerous. In residential homes, nails often protrude down through the plywood subroofing and can cause painful puncture wounds or lacerations in the head and neck. Furthermore, most home attics are not floored; a misstep can drop you through the ceiling of the room below, or leave you with two legs straddling a ceiling joist (ouch!). Fiberglass insulation can irritate your skin, eyes, and respiratory tract, or cause more serious health problems, and you face shock hazards from electrical lines.

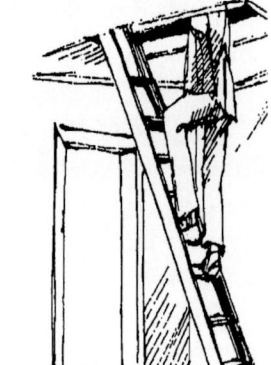

Ladders leading to attics are frequently broken and dangerous

Precautions in Attics

- Wear coveralls, gloves, hard hat, and any other personal protective equipment that you think might be necessary.
- Make sure the attic ladder is safe before using it.
- Disturb insulation as little as possible, particularly blown-in and/or loose insulation in an attic (see *Fiberglass Insulation*).
- Avoid disturbing bird or bat droppings (see *Bird and Bat Roosts*).
- Use a respirator whenever power-spraying or power-dusting, or if you think that there might be any airborne substances (fiberglass threads, vermiculite insulation, etc.) that you do not want to breathe.
- Carry a good flashlight with strong batteries.
- Shine your flashlight on each area of the attic *before* entering it.
- Move slowly and watch where you step. Don't get yourself into a tight space that you may have trouble getting out of.
- Look out for loose or dangling electrical lines. Don't touch any cables.
- If the attic is hot, do not enter it without someone to check on you. Be alert to symptoms of heat illness (see *Heat and Cold*).

Attics rarely have good ventilation, so most pesticides you apply pose an inhalation risk. Attics can also be dangerously hot, and you can get cramps, pulled muscles, or a sore back from working and moving hunched over.

There may be wasps, bees, scorpions and other stinging and biting pests in an attic, as well as bats, birds and their droppings, not to mention the occasional raccoon or opossum.

Crawlspaces

It's dark, it's dirty, it's confined, and it's unfamiliar, yet technicians often work in it. What is it? A crawlspace, of course. Working here can be unpleasant and, to some extent, hazardous. Think about the hazards present in some crawlspaces:

- You can bump your head on pipes, beams, nails, etc.
- You can cut or scrape yourself on broken glass and other debris as you crawl on your belly.
- You can get cramps, pulled muscles, or a sore back from working and moving hunched over.
- In apartment building crawlspaces, in particular, you may be crawling through soil contaminated with old sewage spills from backups or broken pipes.
- You may be crawling through soil contaminated with disease organisms (see sections on *Hookworm* and *Tetanus*).

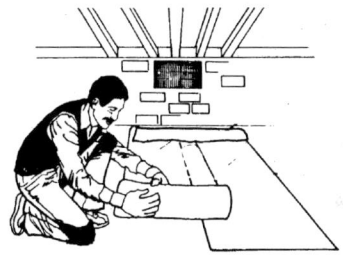

Crawlspaces can be confined, unpleasant, and hazardous places to work

- You may face shock hazards from electrical lines, particularly in wet crawlspaces.
- There may be fleas, spiders, snakes, and other pests to bite or sting you.
- You could surprise a cornered animal such as a raccoon or skunk.
- You could inhale toxicants of various sorts such as pesticide vapors, asbestos, fungal spores, or allergens.
- You risk exposure to bloodborne pathogens such as HIV and hepatitis from the syringes discarded by illegal drug users (see *Bloodborne Pathogens*).

Pest Control Technician Safety Manual

Precautions in Crawlspaces

Before you enter a particular crawlspace, assess the hazards you might face and take action to protect yourself from them. (Many of these hazards are discussed elsewhere in this manual.) Use common sense and your safety training.

- Wear coveralls, gloves, hard hat, and any other personal protective equipment that you think might be necessary.
- Use a respirator if you suspect that the crawl is dusty, or if you think that there might be any airborne substances that you do not want to breathe.
- Carry a good flashlight with strong batteries.
- Shine your flashlight on each area of the crawlspace *before* entering it.
- Move slowly. Don't get yourself into a tight space that you may have trouble getting out of.
- Make sure someone knows that you are going to enter a crawlspace, particularly a tight one.
- Look out for loose or dangling electrical lines. Don't touch any cables, particularly in a wet crawlspace.
- After you leave the crawl, remove any potential contaminants by taking off and bagging your coveralls and gloves, and washing up.

Applying Pesticides in Attics and Crawlspaces

Attics, crawlspaces, and other areas with restricted space and poor ventilation (elevator pits, dumpsters, trash rooms, etc.) pose special hazards to technicians. The concentration of pesticide in the air during application is much higher than

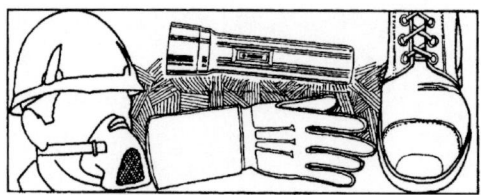

Use adequate personal protective equipment (PPE) when working inside a crawlspace

during application in open, well-ventilated rooms. Working in a restricted space also increases the risk of skin exposure to pesticides from splashback of liquids and dusts, crawling through pesticide already applied, or accidentally touching treated surfaces.

Tight, poorly-ventilated spaces are often hot, further increasing airborne residues through increased volatility, while perspiration and high temperature speed up skin absorption of many pesticides (see also *Confined Spaces*).

> ### *Safety Precautions When Applying Pesticides*
> To minimize your risk of pesticide exposure in poorly-ventilated spaces follow these guidelines:
> - Wear a respirator, eye protection, gloves, lightweight spray suit (or at least coveralls with long sleeves), and any other PPE you think necessary.
> - Increase the ventilation, if possible, by opening windows or vents, or by using fans to bring in fresh air. (Make sure, however, that the increased ventilation does not make your pesticide drift into occupied areas, or get taken up by the ventilation system and recirculate through the building.)
> - Begin your treatment at the point furthest away and work back to your exit point. Avoid walking or crawling through the pesticide you have applied.
> - Avoid working inside a restricted space when the temperature is too high for comfort.
> - Make sure others know where you are and what you are doing. Work with a partner whenever possible.
> - Do not power-dust an attic if you suspect there may be asbestos-containing insulation (see *Asbestos*).

Key Points to Remember—Attics and Crawlspaces

- √ *Before you enter an attic or crawlspace, assess the hazards you might face and take proper action to protect yourself.*
- √ *Make sure someone knows you are entering the space.*
- √ *Wear coveralls, gloves, hard hat, and other personal protective equipment that you think is necessary.*
- √ *Carry a good flashlight with strong batteries, and check out each area before entering it.*
- √ *Make sure the attic ladder is safe before using it.*
- √ *Use a respirator and other PPE whenever power-spraying or power-dusting in locations with poor ventilation (see Power-Dusting and Power-Spraying).*
- √ *Begin your treatment at the point furthest away and work back to your exit point.*
- √ *Don't touch any cables or loose or dangling electrical lines.*

BIRD AND BAT ROOSTS

Certain disease-causing organisms grow in bird or bat droppings. A thick layer of droppings from years of roosting provides a rich, nutritious brew, especially for the disease fungi that cause histoplasmosis ("histo") and cryptococcosis ("crypto"). Histoplasmosis is often found in bird and bat droppings on soil under roosts; cryptococcosis more often in pigeon droppings at elevated roost sites. Both diseases are spread when droppings are disturbed during building renovation or during cleanup of the droppings under an old roost site. After the disturbance, the spores or vegetative cells float in the air by the millions. Workers nearby, or others downwind, may inhale them into their lungs and become infected. Bird droppings are most hazardous when they are dry and can become airborne as a fine dust.

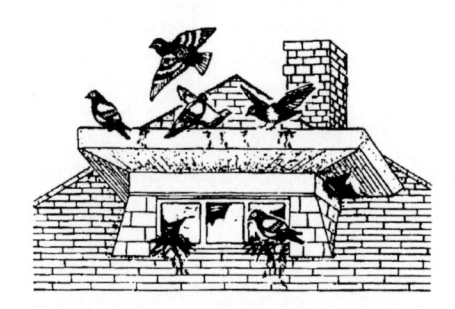

Dry bird and bat droppings pose risk of a number of diseases and other health impacts

When infected with one of these diseases, most people show no symptoms or, at the most, mild flu-like symptoms. But if someone breathes a high concentration of spores or cells, or is particularly susceptible to the disease, the infection can become serious, sometimes even deadly.

There is a lesser known but also dangerous health threat associated with bird roosts. Allergenic hypersensitivity pneumonitis is a potentially disabling lung disease, not caused by an infectious agent, but by an allergic reaction to airborne debris from bird feathers, droppings, and other bird proteins. Experts estimate that from one to five percent of individuals exposed to bird proteins (antigens) will develop symptoms.

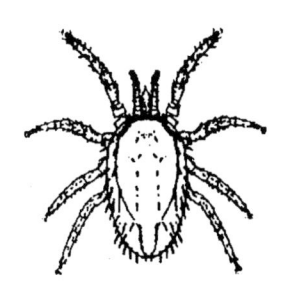

Certain bird mites, bat bugs, and other ectoparasites of birds and bats can bite people, including technicians working near their nest sites.

When working around bat roosts, you also need to think about rabies. If you are bitten, scratched, or have direct contact with a bat, take immediate precautions against rabies, which should include capturing or killing the bat for testing (if possible), cleaning any wound, and seeing a physician for rabies vaccination. See rabies discussions in *Wildlife* and in *Vaccinations*.

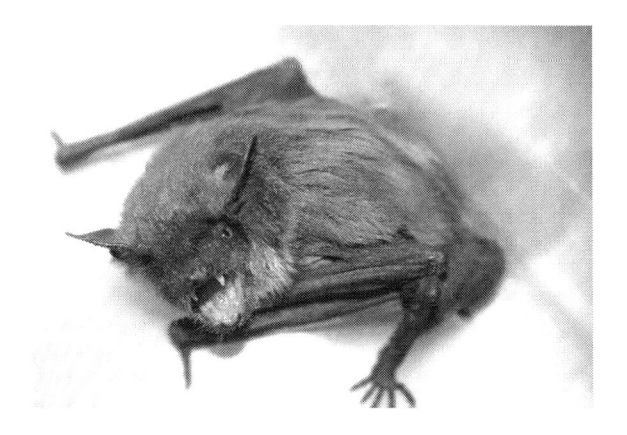

Bird mites can attack people...even technicians

Bats can transmit rabies through bites, scratches, and other direct contact

photo © Michelle Hamel/iStockphoto

Precautions Around Bird and Bat Roosts

Follow the precautions listed below to protect yourself and others when you work in old bird and bat roosts, especially if you are removing accumulations of bird droppings.

- Wear a respirator equipped with an HE (high efficiency) filter, (color-coded magenta or red-purple) that can filter particles down to 0.3 microns, or a supplied-air respirator. Dust masks are not adequate. Any N100, R100, or P100 filter is classified as an HE filter.
- Wear disposable protective gloves, hat, coveralls, eye protection, and booties. (Be careful about heat illness when wearing this protective clothing in warm weather—see *Heat and Cold*).
- Turn off any and all HVAC systems.
- Gently wet down the droppings to keep spores from becoming airborne.
- Put wet droppings into sealed plastic garbage bags and wet the outside of the bags.
- When finished, and while still wearing the respirator, remove the protective clothing and place it inside a plastic garbage bag. Only when you have the clothing bagged should you remove your respirator.
- Dispose of the trash bags that contain the droppings. In most areas, disposal should be permitted through standard trash pickup (bird droppings are EPA-classified as livestock waste, not hazardous waste).
- Put nondisposable work clothing and the respirator in plastic bags. Both should be decontaminated and washed before they are used again.

Bird or Bat Roost Health Warning

If you develop flu-like symptoms days or even weeks after disturbing material in a bird or bat roost, and the illness worsens rather than subsides after a few days, seek medical care. Tell the health care provider about your possible exposure to histoplasmosis and cryptococcosis.

Key Points to Remember—Bird and Bat Roosts

- √ **The disease organisms causing histoplasmosis and cryptococcosis may grow where bird or bat droppings accumulate.**
- √ **Both diseases are spread when droppings are disturbed during building renovation or during cleanup of droppings under an old roost site.**
- √ **Bird and bat droppings are most dangerous when they are dry and become airborne as a fine dust that can be inhaled.**
- √ **You must follow special precautions to protect yourself and others nearby when working in old bird and bat roosts.**
- √ **If you experience persistent flu-like symptoms after disturbing a roost, consult a physician.**
- √ **Ectoparasites and rabid bats are other concerns when working in bird and bat roosts.**

BLOODBORNE PATHOGENS

Blood, body fluids, and medical waste may contain pathogens—agents that cause disease. In hospitals, medical laboratories, nursing homes, and the homes of those under medical care, these pathogens, usually called "bloodborne pathogens," are serious hazards to those working in the area. In medical facilities, warning signs are often placed on the doors of high risk areas (learn to recognize them!)...but not always.

Universal Biohazard Sign

The universal biohazard sign is placed on doors and on equipment (such as incubators, freezers, animal cages, and medical waste boxes) to warn you that a room or a piece of equipment may contain a possible human pathogen. If you see this sign, do not open equipment or enter a room unless you have been authorized to do so.

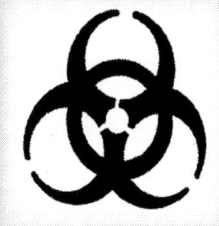

Blood

Exposure to blood can be hazardous to your health. The infectious pathogens it may contain include human immunodeficiency virus (HIV), which can cause AIDS, and hepatitis B virus, which can cause a wide range of liver problems.

Why should you worry about the hazards associated with blood? You may work in hospitals, nursing homes, dental offices, medical labs, and other facilities where blood, used bandages, contaminated needles, human tissues, and other potentially infectious materials are commonplace. (More than one technician has looked into a stainless steel bucket in an emergency room and been shocked to find pieces of skin and parts of human organs.)

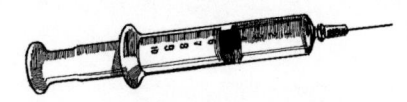

Used needles may contain bloodborne pathogens

You may work in housing where blood-contaminated needles from both legal and illegal drug use are discarded in crawlspaces, basements, under beds, left in sofas, or even left out in the open. Or you may someday have to give emergency first aid to someone who is injured. In all these cases you could be exposed to "bloodborne pathogens" that put you at risk. To protect yourself when working in sites where you might be exposed to bloodborne pathogens, you should:

(1) Become familiar with bloodborne diseases and how they're transmitted.
(2) Wear the proper safety equipment for the site. If you might be exposed to bloodborne pathogens, you should wear disposable gloves, and sometimes two pair to protect you if the outer pair should tear. If there's any chance that blood or bodily fluids could be splashed or become airborne, you may also need to wear goggles, a respirator, or other personal protective equipment.
(3) Avoid needlesticks. Never reach into areas where you can't see such as trash cans, under sofa cushions or mattresses, etc. (see *Needlesticks*).
(4) Never touch medical waste, bandages, blood or bodily fluids, or contaminated laundry.
(5) If you are unsure whether you should be entering a medical or laboratory area... don't.

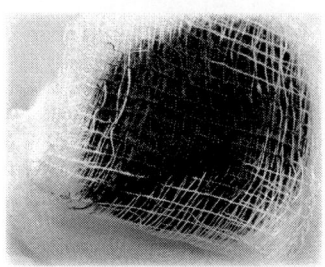

Never touch medical waste, bandages, and other blood-contaminated items

(6) When giving first aid, avoid contact with blood, wear gloves if possible, and use a mouth mask if performing CPR.
(7) Consider getting vaccinated for the hepatitis B virus, which is transmitted by infected blood (see *Vaccinations*).

Bloodborne Pathogens and PPE

You may need to use personal protective equipment (PPE) to protect yourself from bloodborne pathogens. Here are some precautions to follow:

- Remove PPE after it becomes contaminated, and before leaving the work area.
- Wash hands immediately <u>before</u>, and then <u>after,</u> removal of gloves or other PPE.
- Place used PPE in appropriate containers for storage, laundering, decontamination, or disposal.
- Wear appropriate gloves when it can be reasonably anticipated that there may be hand contact with blood or other potentially infected materials, and when handling or touching contaminated items or surfaces; replace gloves if torn, punctured, contaminated, or if their ability to function as a barrier is compromised.
- Utility gloves may be decontaminated for reuse only if they do not show any signs of cracking, peeling, tearing, puncturing, or deterioration.
- Never wash or decontaminate disposable gloves for reuse.
- Wear appropriate face and eye protection when splashes, sprays, spatters, or droplets of blood or other potentially infected materials pose a hazard to the eyes, nose, or mouth.
- Remove immediately, or as soon as you can, any garment contaminated by blood or other potentially infected materials, in such a way as to avoid contact with the garment's outside surface.

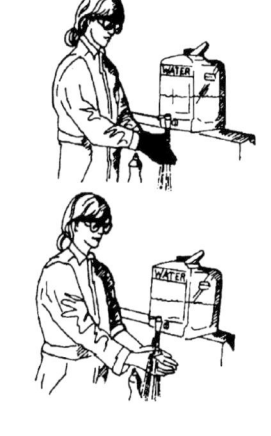

Wash hands immediately before, and then after, removal of gloves or other PPE

See also *Hospitals, Needlesticks,* and *Tuberculosis (TB)*.

> *What to Do if Exposed to a Potential Bloodborne Pathogen*
> If you contact blood or bodily fluids, take immediate action:
>
> **If your skin is broken**—Vigorously scrub the contaminated area for 15 minutes with an iodine solution and large amounts of water. If an iodine solution is not available, scrub with soap (antibacterial if available) and water for 15 minutes.
>
> **If your skin is not broken**—Vigorously scrub the contaminated area for 15 minutes with soap (antibacterial if available) and water.
>
> **For eyes and mucous membranes**—Irrigate eyes and mucous membranes for 15 minutes with normal saline solution or with clean water.
>
> **Then**—Call your supervisor and seek medical attention within one hour of exposure. Quick medical attention may prevent serious illness.

Key Points to Remember—Bloodborne Pathogens

- √ Blood may contain bloodborne pathogens such as HIV and hepatitis B virus.
- √ Exposure to blood or medical waste can be hazardous to your health.
- √ You could be exposed to bloodborne pathogens in medical facilities, or when giving first aid, or where there is illegal drug use.
- √ Wear the proper safety equipment if you might be exposed to bloodborne pathogens.
- √ Remove any garment contaminated by blood or body fluids, and avoid contact with the outer surface.
- √ Never touch medical waste, bandages, blood or bodily fluids, or contaminated laundry.
- √ When giving first aid, avoid contact with blood, wear gloves if possible, and use a mouth mask if performing CPR.
- √ If you do have accidental contact with blood or bodily fluids, immediately wash with soap and water, flush out eyes or mouth with running water, and seek medical attention.

COMPRESSED GAS CYLINDERS

Pressurized fumigants and other compressed gas cylinders used in pest control can be hazardous. Not only are there risks from the contents (fumigants, insecticides, propane, etc.), but there are also risks from bursting or other catastrophic pressure release. Safe handling of compressed gas cylinders is regulated by OSHA, DOT, EPA (through labeling), as well as state agencies in many states. Safe handling directions are usually based on the guidelines of the Compressed Gas Association, and typically include the following:

- Keep the safety valve protection bonnet and/or safety cap on the cylinder when it is not in use.
- Store and transport cylinders in an upright position.
- Do not strike or heat the valve.
- Do not suspend or lift the cylinder by its valve.
- Do not unload the cylinder with rope slings, hooks, or tongs.
- Secure cylinders in a rack or to a wall to prevent tipping.
- Transport cylinders over short distances using a hand truck, fork truck, or similar device to which the cylinder can be secured.
- Handle cylinders gently, do not drop them, bump them, slide them, or drag them.
- Do not transport cylinders within closed vehicles that have a common airspace for cylinders, driver, and passengers.
- Close valve tightly after use, even if you believe the cylinder is empty.
- Inspect cylinders to make sure they are not damaged, leaking, or corroded.
- Follow manufacturer's instructions for returning cylinders.

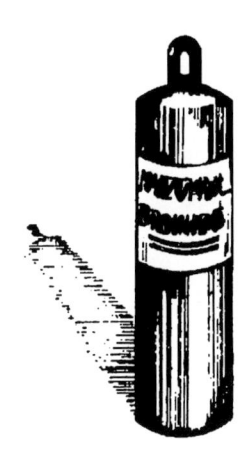

Safe cylinder handling will prevent catastrophic pressure release

Precautions for Compressed Gas Fumigants

Compressed gas fumigants such as Vikane® and methyl bromide require special handling because they are extremely toxic if accidently released near unprotected people. Besides the safety guidelines from the Compressed Gas Association that were listed earlier, follow these special precautions for fumigants packaged in pressurized cylinders:

- Store cylinders outside if possible, and protect them from the elements.
- If stored inside, the storage area should be isolated from workplaces and offices, and have proper ventilation.
- If cylinders are stored in an enclosed area without proper ventilation, the area needs to be checked regularly for leaking gas with proper fumigant detection equipment (Interscan® gas analyzer, Miran® vapor analyzer, Draeger® tubes or other gas detector tubes).
- If you find a damaged apron ring (cylinder support skirt), return the cylinder to the distributor.
- If you have the choice, carry fumigants on the fumigation vehicle in side racks rather than rear racks because rear-end collisions are more common.
- Always have a SCBA (self-contained breathing apparatus) and valve wrench available.

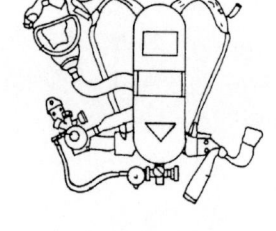

Always have a SCBA and valve wrench available

graphic from SIRI UVM

A Leaking Fumigant Cylinder Is An Emergency!

- Put on your SCBA.
- Stop the leak if you can do so without delay.
- Whether you have stopped the leak or not, clear everyone out of the area unless they are wearing an SCBA.
- If the leaking cylinder is indoors, and you cannot stop the leak, move the cylinder outside. The more isolated the site is, the better. Have people stay upwind, and evacuate people from nearby downwind sites if there is risk of exposure. Keep them away until the cylinder is empty and there is no risk of gas remaining.
- If a cylinder has a slow leak, but you are not sure from where, apply soapy water to the cylinder, valve, and hose connections. Bubbles will form at the leak site.

Key Points to Remember—Compressed Gas Cylinders

√ **Compressed gas cylinders pose risks from unexpected release of their contents and from bursting or other catastrophic pressure release.**

√ **Your handling of compressed gas cylinders is regulated by OSHA and other agencies.**

√ **If you follow the handling guidelines of the Compressed Gas Association, you can minimize risk of accidental gas release.**

√ **If a fumigant cylinder is leaking, evacuate the area.**

CONFINED SPACES

Imagine yourself stuck in a sewer manhole as the water level rises. Or sinking in stored bulk grain and unable to breathe as the grain closes over your head. Or trapped in an elevator pit as the elevator slowly crushes you. Such thoughts could give you nightmares!

These gruesome examples of "confined spaces" are why the Occupational Safety and Health Administration (OSHA) has special rules for entering a confined space that is particularly hazardous—a "permit-required" confined space.

What is a Permit-Required Confined Space?

Many workplaces contain spaces that are "confined," meaning that you may have to work while cramped, restricted or contorted, or else you must squeeze through a small opening to enter. A crawlspace is a confined space.

But if you add an additional hazard such as asphyxiation, entrapment, toxic gases, crush injuries, fire or explosion, then that space becomes a "permit-required" confined space. Examples of permit-required confined spaces in pest control include grain storage bins and sewers (see box next page).

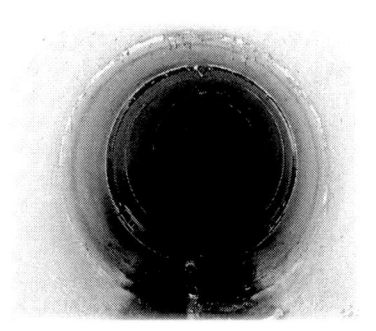

Many workplaces contain spaces that are confined AND hazardous

Storm drain photo USGS

Pest Control Technician Safety Manual

> ### Examples of Permit-Required Confined Spaces in Pest Control
>
> Grain storage bin • Silo • Bulk material hopper
> Elevator pit • Ship hold • Certain grain rail cars
> Sewer manhole • Storm drain vault • Utility vault

Before you can enter such a permit-required confined space, you must comply with a long list of OSHA rules. The first and most obvious is that you must first obtain a permit signed by an "entry supervisor." You must follow a written program specific to that site, and have been trained for entering such spaces. Depending on the hazards at the site, there might need to be air monitoring and ventilation equipment, a stand-by rescue team, rescue equipment (ladders, hoists), isolation of the space (lockout/tagout, police tape), and special personal protective equipment.

Pest control companies often avoid the complications of OSHA requirements by (1) training technicians to recognize a permit-required confined space, and (2) having a policy that technicians may not enter any permit-required confined space.

Whole Grain Storage and Processing

In some areas of the country, PMPs control pests in and around bulk stored whole grains. Examples include silos, bulk storage bins and hoppers, ship holds, and grain rail cars.

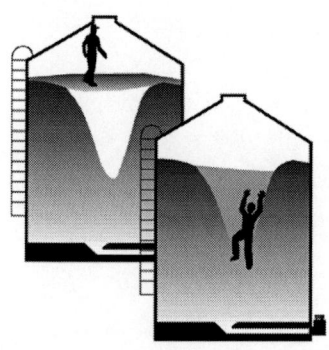

Grain can act like quicksand to pull you under
NDSU Extension Service

Look inside a full grain bin. At first glance, it doesn't seem dangerous. But don't be fooled, and don't even think about walking on the grain without proper equipment and training. People die each year entrapped in grain.

The grain surface that looks so solid can fool you. Grain can act like quicksand to pull you under. You can be completely engulfed in grain in 8 seconds and suffocate in a matter of minutes. Even if you are not completely engulfed, carbon dioxide generated by grain can suffocate you at the surface. If you sink only to your waist, you still won't be able to pull yourself out of the grain; a rescue team will be necessary.

Grain bridges also form in stored grain. Since grain is emptied from the bottom, a void forms below the crusted surface (the bridge), which looks solid but can suddenly collapse, burying you under thousands of pounds of grain.

There are two other entrapment hazards in stored grain. Grain can set up in a large mass against the bin wall in a partially empty bin. When it is disturbed, it can cascade down like an avalanche and bury workers below. Also, never enter a bin, grain rail car, truck, wagon box, or auger pit where grain is actively flowing out, even if the grain is shallow. As grain flows out of the holding area, it creates a suction action so strong that a person cannot swim, climb, or walk against it and escape. The victim will be pulled under very quickly with no time to react.

Because of these hazards, grain storage facilities are usually considered to be permit-required confined spaces, requiring safety harnesses and equipment, rescue team/partner, respirator, and other safety practices and equipment detailed in a written confined spaces program.

Sewers, Storm Drains, Vaults

A sewer is considered by OSHA to be a permit-required confined space because you may face the following hazards when you are inside:

(1) You can be engulfed and trapped if water or sewage suddenly floods the sewer system.
(2) You may be exposed to toxic gases, particularly hydrogen sulfide.
(3) Other gases, such as methane (sewer gas), can cause a fire or explosion.
(4) The air you are breathing may be deficient in oxygen (below about 20%), which could cause you to lose consciousness.

Most technicians should not enter sewer manholes. Most pest control work (rats, cockroaches) can be done from the surface anyway. An exception might be a technician doing work for a municipality or for a large food processing facility. He or she may, on occasion, enter sewers to place rodent baits, remove dead rats, etc., but only if both the owner of the sewer (the sewer

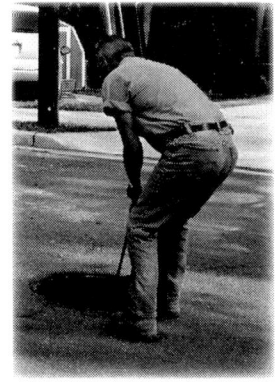

Sewers, manholes, and vaults are "permit-required" confined spaces

service authority or the food processing plant) and the pest control company have written permit-required confined spaces programs in place and follow a long list of other rules.

> ### ALERT—Confined Spaces Rescue
> Over 50 percent of workers who die in confined spaces are attempting to rescue other workers. This type of rescue is challenging and dangerous. Do not try to rescue a coworker trapped in a permit-required confined space unless you are trained and equipped to do so. Instead, call the proper rescue team or 911. Otherwise, your first unplanned rescue could be your last. *(OSHA photo.)*

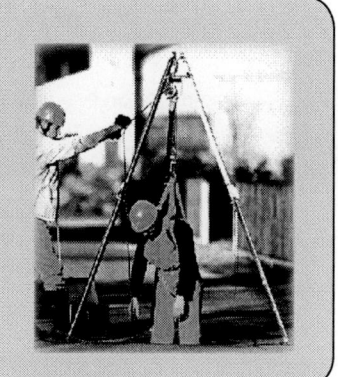

OSHA Definitions Related to Confined Spaces

"A confined space has limited or restricted means of entry or exit, is large enough for an employee to enter and perform assigned work, and is not designed for continuous occupancy by the employee. These spaces may include, but are not limited to, underground vaults, tanks, storage bins, pits and diked areas, vessels, and silos."

"A permit-required confined space is one that meets the definition of confined space and has one or more of these characteristics: (1) contains or has the potential to contain a hazardous atmosphere, (2) contains a material that has the potential for engulfing an entrant, (3) has an internal configuration that might cause an entrant to be trapped or asphyxiated by inwardly converging walls or by a floor that slopes downward and tapers to a smaller cross section, and/or (4) contains any other recognized serious safety or health hazards."

Key Points to Remember—Confined Spaces

- √ **OSHA requires a permit for entering certain confined spaces in the workplace because they are especially hazardous.**
- √ **Sewers, storm drains, manhole vaults, grain bins, and elevator pits are examples of permit-required confined spaces.**

- √ **Before anyone can enter a permit-required confined space, a long list of OSHA-mandated requirements must be met.**
- √ **Most technicians will never need to enter a permit-required confined space.**
- √ **Do not enter a permit-required confined space unless (1) you have been authorized by the owner or operator to enter it and (2) you have been trained in the special safety requirements of permit-space entry.**
- √ **Do not try to rescue a coworker trapped in a permit-required confined space unless you are trained and equipped to do so.**

DRIVING AND VEHICLE SAFETY

Three workers are killed every day — more than a thousand each year — in job-related traffic accidents. Workers fatally injured in vehicle crashes are mostly male (93 percent); are aged 25 to 54 (70 percent); are drivers (76 percent) as opposed to pedestrians or vehicle passengers; and *most are not using any type of safety restraint (62 percent)*.

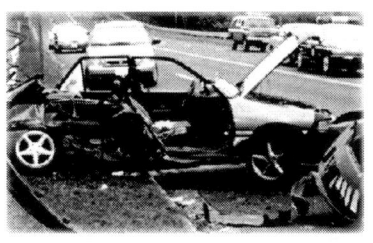

Over 60 percent of workers killed in crashes were not wearing seat belts
National Highway Traffic Safety Administration

General Safe Driving Guidelines

You probably spend a lot of your day driving. How much of that time do you actually think about driving? Chances are you're more worried about arriving at your next job on time or whether your flashlight is sitting in the kitchen you just left. The question is, will you react quickly enough in an emergency to avoid an accident? Be safe. Drive defensively and follow these guidelines:

- Use seat belts at all times. Make sure there's a seat belt for each passenger and that passengers are belted in.
- Don't drive if you're too tired to think or react clearly, or if you're so sleepy that you might doze off.
- Be careful when taking prescription and over-the-counter drugs. Some can leave you drowsy and uncoordinated.

- Do not drive under the influence of alcohol or drugs.
- Drive defensively.
- Always drive within the speed limit. Don't feel you have to rush to your next stop.
- Scan ahead. At turnpike speeds it takes 20 seconds to spot and prepare for trouble ahead, like fog or stopped traffic. At the first sign of something out of the ordinary, slow down, check the position of vehicles near you, and turn on lights or flashers.
- Check behind your vehicle before backing in residential areas (see guidelines under *Backing*)
- Scan your mirrors. Check your rearview and side mirrors every few seconds to note the position of vehicles around you in case you have to change lanes fast to avoid having an accident.
- Keep your distance. Allow the driver in front of you enough space to stop, change lanes, or turn. If you're being tailgated, protect yourself by giving turn signals well in advance--and avoid sudden stops. Change lanes or slow down so that the tailgater will pass (see *The "Two-Second Rule"*).
- Use your signals. Signal early, well before your turn.
- Use care at intersections. About 40% of all city auto accidents occur at intersections, often because one driver tries to beat another across an intersection rather than yield the right-of-way.

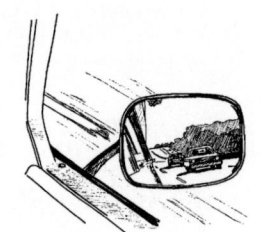

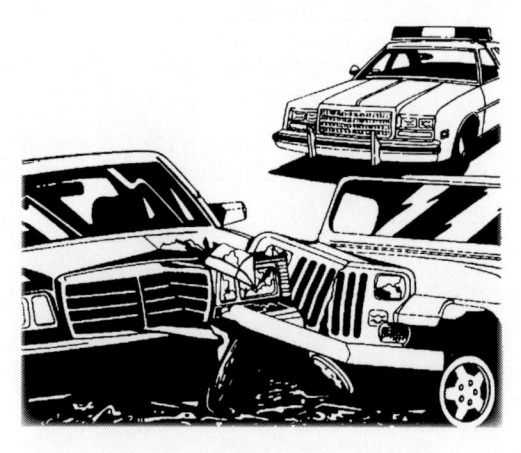

Scan your mirrors every few seconds

Be safe by driving defensively

- Consider the weather. Rain, snow, and ice make it more difficult to stop or turn. (Four-wheel drive and front-wheel drive vehicles stop no faster that rear-wheel drive vehicles.) A road will be most slippery just after rain begins because the rainwater mixes with oil on the road surface. In cold weather, bridges freeze before roads. Be wary of "black ice" anytime the temperature is below freezing and the road looks wet. Slow down in fog.
- Drive gently. Do not be aggressive. Nowadays, traffic arguments sometimes escalate to fights, battles between vehicles, or can even end with a bullet.
- Make sure your vehicle is properly maintained (see *Inspection and Maintenance*).
- Be familiar with and know how to operate your vehicle's safety features such as antilock brakes, emergency flashers, daytime running lights. Make sure air bags have not been disabled.
- In case of a vehicle breakdown, have the appropriate flares, reflective triangles, and cones to alert traffic.

Special Rollover Precautions for Trucks and Vans

Vehicle rollovers are not new but they have received more attention lately as the proportion of SUVs, trucks, and vans has increased. Rollovers are almost always single-vehicle crashes and can be prevented. Rollovers typically occur when a driver has to suddenly swerve to avoid an obstacle or a stopped car in the road, or when the driver accidentally veers off the road due to excessive speed, fatigue, inattentiveness, or drug or alcohol use.

Although rollovers are a relatively rare type of crash, they have a higher death rate than some other types of accidents. One of every three passenger vehicle deaths occurs in a rollover. Because of this high death rate, many new vehicles, especially SUVs, are now equipped with anti-rollover technology such as electronic stability control. By 2012 most new vehicles sold in the U.S. will have to be equipped with such technology.

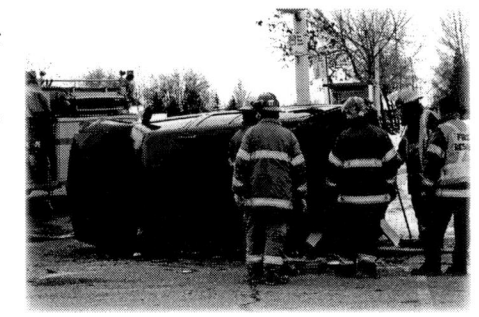

Rollovers are almost always single-vehicle crashes and can be prevented.

Photo © Don Wilkie/iStockphoto

Any vehicle can roll over, but light trucks and vans are more likely to do so. This is because these vehicles have a higher center of gravity and some also tend to "oversteer" with the rear of the vehicle sliding outward. Here are some guidelines for preventing rollover from the AAA Foundation for Traffic Safety and State Farm Insurance.

Load Your Vehicle Properly

Distribute pesticide containers, pumps, sprayers and other items to maintain a weight balance inside. Your vehicle's owner's manual has guidelines on distributing the load and will tell you the maximum safe weight load for the vehicle.

Be Especially Careful of Roof Loads

If you carry ladders or other items on your roof, you raise the center of gravity even more and increase your risk of vehicle rollover. If you can transport items inside the vehicle instead, do so.

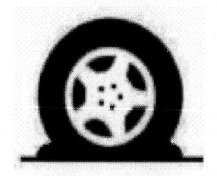

Keep Tires in Good Shape

Tires that are worn or are improperly inflated are common causes of vehicles sliding sideways on wet pavement and rolling over.

Watch Your Speed

Excessive speed is a contributing factor in about 40% of fatal rollovers. Nearly 3 of every 4 fatal rollovers occurs on a rural road with a posted speed limit of 55 mph or higher. The faster you're driving, the less reaction time you have, and that increases the chances that you will steer or brake too sharply causing a rollover.

Know How to Correct

If your vehicle accidentally veers off of the road, don't react too suddenly. Avoid "panic-steering" and overcorrection. Slow down gradually and ease the vehicle back onto the roadway. Sudden steering maneuvers on soft surfaces are a major cause of rollovers.

Buckle Up

About three-quarters of people killed in rollovers were not wearing their seatbelts!

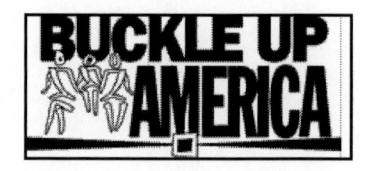

Vehicle Accidents and Failing Eyes

Older drivers have fewer accidents on average than younger drivers. It appears, however, that vehicle safety is related to vision clarity in older drivers. Eyes undergo a number of age-related changes. Some of the most common are (1) inability to adapt from light to darkness, (2) glare sensitivity, and (3) lack of contrast. A research study showed that the incidence of traffic fatalities was significantly lower (10-12 percent) in states that require vision tests in drivers over 60 than in states that don't require such testing.

Whatever your state's policy, if you are an older technician, have your eyes checked regularly to detect problems early. Many age-related vision problems can be corrected. Others require work changes to minimize hazards; for example, driving only during daylight hours.

The "Two-Second Rule"

"Rear-ender" accidents happen more than eight times as often as any other type of collision. The average driver's reaction time is 3/4 of a second. That means that at just 40 mph, you'll travel 44 feet just trying to get to the brake pedal. In all, you'll eat up about 120 feet from the time you see a problem until you've stopped your car or truck. Add weather conditions or a loaded vehicle and you increase that distance significantly.

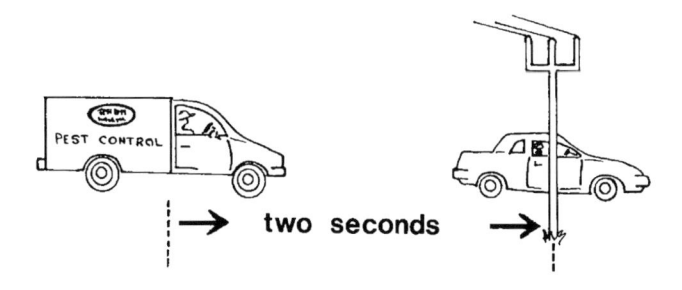

If your vehicle passes the same landmark before you count "one thousand and one, one thousand and two," you are too close!

Follow the "two-second rule" of driving: When the car ahead of you passes a road sign or other landmark, start counting, "one thousand and one, one thousand and two." If your car passes the same landmark before you finish counting, you're too close and may not be able to stop safely. At turnpike speeds, in bad road conditions, or with a tailgater on your rear, increase your following distance to four seconds.

Dealing with Tailgaters

No matter what speed you're driving, it seems there's always somebody riding on your tail, like a shadow. You speed up, he speeds up. You slow down, he slows down. And he won't pass. What should you do?

First of all, if the right lane is open, change lanes. Otherwise, gradually reduce your speed. By allowing extra space in front of you, you'll encourage the tailgater to pass. If he doesn't, you've given yourself extra room, allowing more time for you (and the tailgater) to come to a stop.

Avoid Distractions

Life is full of distractions. Driving shouldn't be. During the few seconds that you take your eyes off of the road to look at a map or pick up a hamburger, you may miss seeing the driver in front of you slam on his brakes. According to the National Highway Traffic Safety Administration (NHTSA), almost 80 percent of crashes and 65 percent of near misses occur within three seconds of some form of driver distraction.

Is This the Right Exit?

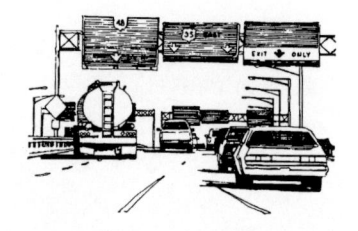

Plan your route *before* you leave your last account. Don't fumble with a map while driving; pull off of the road to read it. If you must consult a map while underway, place it in a dash-mounted clipboard or in some other location in front of you where you can quickly glance at it and still keep both hands on the wheel.

Plan your route <u>before</u> you leave

"Is That for Here or to Go"?

Don't eat and drive. It can be too distracting. Say you're driving to a one o'clock account, eating a hamburger. You drip ketchup onto your pants. Momentary panic trying to clean up the mess. You're no longer looking at the road. When you glance up again, you suddenly see...

Besides the distraction, there's another good reason not to eat while driving. When you grab a fast food lunch to eat in your truck, you're less likely to stop and wash your hands first. You may transfer pesticide residues from your hands to your mouth or your food. Further, even if you have washed, there could be pesticide residue on your steering wheel, or on the seat where you're about to set that sandwich.

Stay Off That Cell Phone

More and more accidents are occurring when drivers lose concentration while using a cell phone. A study by researchers at the University of Toronto estimated that a driver using a cell phone increased his or her risk of an accident by more than four times, a rate equivalent to intoxication. Using a cell phone is a potentially dangerous distraction while driving. In some states and cities it is illegal. Hang up and drive, or stop and phone.

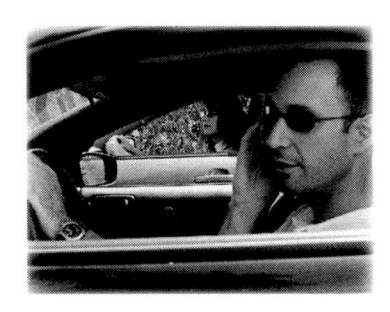

Cell phone use increases accident risk 4X

Photo H. Schmaedeke U.S. Census Bureau

Writing on the Road Isn't Right

The best time to write up your service visit is while it's still fresh in your mind and *before* you get behind the wheel. If you can't take the time then, make a few reminder notes and complete your paperwork at the next stop or at the end of the day. Don't fill out service tickets or other paperwork while driving. Your reports need to be accurate and complete, which is less likely if you're thinking about driving and writing at the same time.

Backing

Backing a vehicle, especially a truck, is always dangerous, because you cannot see very well. Avoid backing whenever you can. Here are some guidelines to follow:

- When you park, try to park so you will be able to pull forward when you leave.
- Walk back and look at your path before backing.
- Back slowly.
- Back and turn towards the driver's side when possible.
- Use a helper if possible.

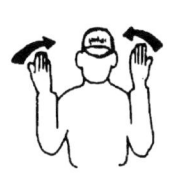

A helper can signal when it is safe to back

Requirements For DOT-Regulated Vehicles

If your company vehicle is Department of Transportation (DOT)-regulated, you must comply with special federal and state regulations. (Note: If your vehicle has DOT numbers displayed on each side, then it is subject to DOT regulations.)

Roadside Inspections

DOT-regulated commercial vehicles must be well maintained and are required to carry certain markings and equipment. DOT-regulated vehicles are subject to roadside inspections either by a state trooper or motor carrier inspector. There are five levels of roadside inspection that can include, in addition to a safety check of the vehicle, required paperwork such as driver's medical examiner's certificate, logbook, fuel tax permit, and more.

Display of DOT Numbers and Company Name

The Federal Motor Carrier Safety Administration (FMCSA) issues a U.S. DOT number to each company. All commercial vehicles in a company receive the same number which is preceded by the acronym USDOT. The number must be displayed on each side of the truck or car and must contrast in color with the background so that it can be seen for a distance of 50 feet. Your company's commercial vehicles must display the legal name of your company in contrasting colors that can be seen from 50 feet away.

Each state will have specific rules regarding commercial vehicle markings and license plates, which may be different, and states may require an additional road use fuel tax sticker.

Required Safety Equipment

Commercial vehicles must be equipped with the following:
- Fire extinguishers. One National Fire Protection Association extinguisher rated 5 B:C or above, or two extinguishers rated 4 B:C or above. A vehicle that is placarded for carrying hazardous materials must have a fire extinguisher with a minimum rating of 10 B:C. Fire extinguishers must be securely mounted on the vehicle, yet must be easily accessible.
- Spare fuses for brake lights.
- Emergency flares or 3 red emergency triangles. Since liquid-burning flares have a limited life, the vehicle must carry enough to last for an extensive breakdown. Flares are not allowed if the material being transported is

explosive, combustible, or flammable. Reflective emergency triangles can be used in any situation and can be reused.
- Retroreflective tape. All trailers with a GVWR of more than 10,000 pounds and widths of more than 80 inches must be marked with retroreflective tape, also called conspicuity tape, to improve night visibility.

Vehicle Inspections

Each commercial vehicle should have two daily inspections: a pre-trip visual inspection and a post-trip written inspection. The pre-trip inspection assures that the vehicle is in operating condition but no documentation is required. At the end of their shift, drivers must perform a post-trip inspection and complete a Daily Vehicle Inspection Report (DVIR).

A vehicle with deficiencies must be removed from the working fleet until repairs can be made. All repairs must be noted on the DVIR, signed by the person who made the repairs. An annual vehicle inspection is required for all commercial vehicles, including trailers. This inspection form also must be documented and signed.

Vehicle maintenance, repair, and inspection forms must be kept for as long as the vehicle is operated and for 6 months after the vehicle leaves the business.

Vehicle Registration and Plates

The original copy of the vehicle registration and the trailer registration must be kept in the vehicle, and proper license plates mounted and visible.

Inspection and Maintenance

If you have a *Commercial Driver's License* (CDL), U.S. Department of Transportation (DOT) and state rules require that you inspect your vehicle before each trip. The inspection is quite detailed. The primary reason is safety. A vehicle defect uncovered during a pre-trip inspection can prevent an accident later in the day.

Even if you don't have a CDL, a pre-trip inspection of your vehicle is a good safety practice. It will only take a few minutes of your time.

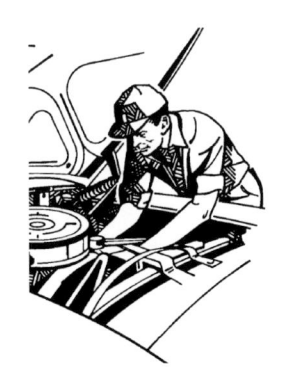

A pre-trip inspection is a required safety practice for commercial drivers

Pest Control Technician Safety Manual

Start your inspection as you approach your vehicle, looking for damage, puddles of fluid, or the vehicle leaning to one side. Systematically check the following systems and items:

Check Engine Compartment

- all fluid levels within proper range
- belts tight and undamaged
- no leaks or visible damage
- no cracked wiring insulation
- steering box/linkage undamaged
- battery charged and secure

Check Inside Cab

- start engine; gauges working
- all controls working normally
- mirrors and windows okay
- all emergency equipment on board
- brakes work properly *(for hydraulic brakes: pump three times then hold for five seconds: pedal should not move)*
- parking brake holds
- shipping papers, permits, etc. on board
- no loose articles
- extra fuses available
- seat belts undamaged

Walk-Around Inspection

Visually check the following items for operation and damage:

- all lights, including turn signals and brake lights
- glass and reflectors
- tires (including spare)
- wheels/rims
- wheel bearings not leaking
- brake drums
- shock absorbers
- suspension (springs/struts)
- axles
- wipers/washers
- splash guards

- cargo and/or tank secure, no leaks
- license plates
- DOT and other markings

Jump-Starting

Jump-starting a car or truck--what's to know? You could do it blindfolded. Don't be too sure. A battery, even one that's "dead," contains concentrated sulfuric acid. That's nasty, corrosive stuff and can cause severe burns if you get it on your skin or in your eyes. On the rare occasion when a battery does explode, acid is sprayed everywhere. If that's not enough, a battery also generates hydrogen gas which is flammable and explosive. If company policy permits you to jump-start a vehicle (and some companies forbid it), follow these safety rules:

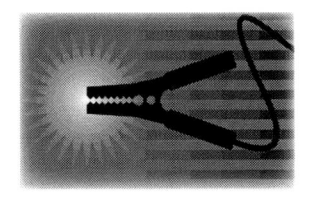

A spark while jump-starting can ignite hydrogen gas at the battery

<small>photo © penfold/iStockphoto</small>

1. Make sure you have a good, well-insulated set of cables. The red clamps are for positive and the black clamps are for negative.
2. To protect your eyes, put on a pair of protective goggles. Remove watches and any metal jewelry that might make an electrical contact. Avoid flames or sparks. Don't smoke.
3. If the booster battery is in another vehicle, make sure that the vehicles are not touching. Turn off unnecessary lights, heater, radio, etc. The voltage of the booster battery and that of the dead battery should be the same.
4. If either battery has filler caps, remove them. Lay a cloth over the open filler holes on both batteries to reduce the explosion hazard.
5. Consult your vehicle owner's manual for the recommended procedure to connect the cables. If you don't have an owner's manual, follow this order: (1) positive cable on the booster battery (2) positive cable on the dead battery (3) negative cable on the booster battery (4) negative cable to a "ground," usually the engine block, on the car with the dead battery.
6. While connecting the cables, be careful not to let the clamps touch each other or anything except the correct terminals or the ground. Don't lean over the battery when making connections.
7. Start the engine in the vehicle with the booster battery. Let it idle a few minutes. Then start the "dead" battery and run the engine at a fast idle speed for several minutes.

8. Disconnect the cables in the reverse order that you connected them: the negative cable first, then the positive cable. Be careful of the fan and moving belts.
9. Replace the battery filler caps and dispose of any rags you were using since they're now contaminated with sulfuric acid.

If you should accidentally get acid on your skin, immediately remove any contaminated clothing. Flush the affected area with plenty of water.

Steer Clear of Static Electricity at Gas Pump

We all know of the warning not to smoke while pumping gas. But static sparks apparently cause far more fires at the pump than does smoking. The static occurs most often by sliding in and out of the car seat during the fueling process. When the driver touches the vehicle body, fuel cap or dispensing nozzle, the static spark can ignite fuel vapors and cause an explosion and fire.

Here are consumer refueling and fuel safety guidelines from the American Petroleum Institute for refueling your vehicle:

- Turn off your vehicle engine. Put your vehicle in park and/or set the emergency brake. Disable or turn off any auxiliary sources of ignition such as a camper or trailer heater, cooking units, or pilot lights.
- Do not smoke, light matches or lighters while refueling at the pump or when using gasoline anywhere else.
- Use only the refueling latch provided on the gasoline dispenser nozzle. Never jam the refueling latch on the nozzle open.
- Do not re-enter your vehicle during refueling. If you cannot avoid re-entering your vehicle, discharge any static build-up BEFORE reaching for the nozzle by touching something metal, such as the vehicle door, with a bare hand (but make the touch away from the nozzle).
- In the unlikely event a static-caused fire occurs when refueling, leave the nozzle in the fill pipe and back away from the vehicle. Notify the station attendant immediately.

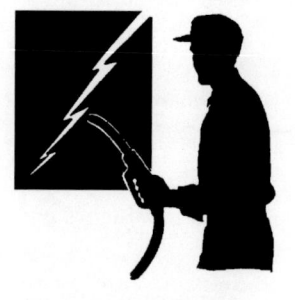

Static sparks cause far more fires at the pump than does smoking

Filling Gas Cans in Vehicles

A fire can also spontaneously ignite if you attempt to fill a portable gasoline container (gas can) on a plastic bed liner in a pickup truck, or in a carpeted car trunk. These fires are caused by the buildup of static electricity. The gasoline flowing into the container generates a static charge that is prevented from grounding by the insulating effect of the truck bed liner or carpet. This static buildup is then discharged to the grounded gasoline dispenser nozzle and may cause a spark and ignite the gasoline. Both ungrounded metal (most hazardous) and plastic gas containers have been involved in these incidents. The problem is resolved by providing a pathway to release the static charge buildup.

Precautions When Filling Gas Cans

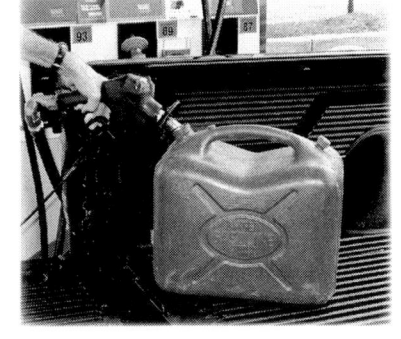

- Do not refill portable gasoline containers while they are inside pickup trucks or cars.
- Remove the containers from the vehicle and place them on the ground at a safe distance from the vehicle. (Placing the container on the ground provides a path to dissipate any static charge.)
- Touch the container with the gas dispenser nozzle before removing the container lid. (This provides another path to dissipate any static charge to the ground.)
- Keep the nozzle in contact with the container inlet when filling. (This dissipates static charge buildup from the flow of gasoline.)
- Manually control the nozzle valve throughout the filling process.
- Fill a portable container slowly to decrease the chance of static electricity buildup and minimize spilling or splattering.

Do not refill portable gasoline containers while they are inside pickup trucks or cars

See discussion of gasoline in *Pesticides and Other Chemicals*.

Pesticides in Vehicles

The pesticides in your vehicle may be in original packaging, in a service container, or ready for application in your spray tank or duster. In all cases, they have to be stored neatly and safely before you hit the road.

Pest Control Technician Safety Manual

- Don't store pesticides in the cab or passenger cabin of your vehicle. First, you want to avoid inhaling pesticide fumes in an enclosed space. Second, even in a minor accident, loose containers in the cab are not going to stay put. Upholstery that is contaminated with pesticides may be impossible to clean.
- Store pesticides in a separate part of the vehicle that can be locked--the covered bed of a truck or a trunk.
- When pesticides are transferred from their original container into a different container or tank, the replacement container must be clearly labeled.
- Pack pesticide containers snugly so that they cannot shift or roll. Make sure to cushion glass containers so that they don't break.
- Containers larger than five gallons (and your compressed air sprayer) should be strapped or tied to the sides of the vehicle, or held in place with blocks or sand bags. Never stack pesticide containers higher than the sides of the truck bed. Don't stack heavy containers on top of lighter ones.
- Containers smaller than five gallons are best stored in a sturdy box, insulated against temperature extremes, and cushioned and compartmentalized to keep containers from bumping against each other. This box should be labeled, secured to the floor, and lockable. Avoid using a cardboard or wooden box since they absorb pesticide odors. A large chest-type cooler that can be padded, secured to the vehicle, and fitted with a hasp lock is a good choice.

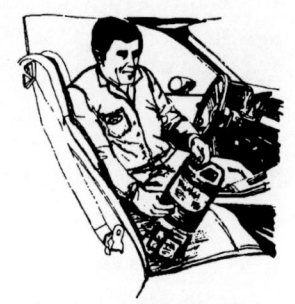

Don't carry pesticides in the cab or in the passenger cabin

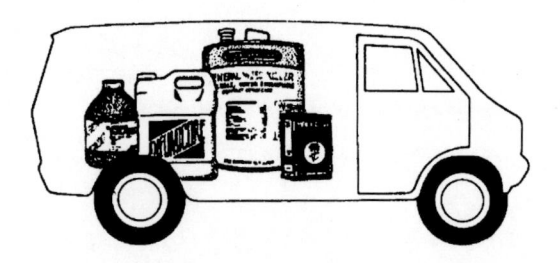

During temperature extremes...either hot or cold...remove chemicals from your vehicle overnight

- Make sure pressurized containers are capped or secured so that an aerosol isn't accidentally released.
- Your vehicle should have an emergency spill control kit, with absorbent material, in case a pesticide container should spill or leak.
- Ideally, the pesticide storage area of your vehicle should be heated in cold weather and cooled in hot weather. Since this is rarely practical, store pesticides in insulated containers in your vehicle. During temperature extremes, remove chemicals from your vehicle overnight or when the vehicle is out of service for long periods.
- If you use your vehicle for personal use, don't allow children or pets to ride with the pesticides, or where pesticides could have been spilled. Don't transport food or feed...or your lunch...in the same compartment with pesticides.
- Wash your steering wheel at least once a week to remove pesticide residues. (Pesticide residues on your hands can be transferred to your steering wheel. Whenever you drive, you'll be re-exposed.)

See also *Pesticides and Other Chemicals*.

Onboard Pesticide Checklist

How pesticides are stored in your vehicle is important, not just for your safety but for the safety of others in case of an accident that could result in a spill. Use the checklist on the next page to see how your vehicle measures up.

Key Points to Remember—Driving and Vehicle Safety

- √ **Use seat belts at all times.**
- √ **Follow the "two-second" rule.**
- √ **Avoid backing whenever you can.**
- √ **Inspect your vehicle before each trip.**
- √ **Load vans and trucks properly and take other precautions to minimize the risk of rollover.**
- √ **Don't store pesticides in the cab or passenger part of your vehicle.**
- √ **Do not refill portable gasoline containers while they are inside pickup trucks or cars.**

Onboard Pesticide Checklist

1. Are you handling pesticide containers properly?
   - Containers properly labeled
   - Containers properly sealed
   - Small containers boxed or secured to avoid sliding or rolling
   - Glass containers cushioned
   - No heavy containers stacked on top of lighter ones
   - Containers kept in insulated coolers during temperature extremes
   - Empty containers properly stored for later triple-rinsing or disposal
   - Sprayer and containers larger than 5-gallons strapped or tied to the sides
   - Not carrying more pesticides than necessary

2. Do you have the necessary safety/spill equipment onboard?
   - Spill control kit (absorbent, bags, rags, police tape, etc.)
   - First aid kit
   - Plastic jug of clean water, labeled "CLEAN WATER"
   - Respirator, goggles, gloves, other PPE
   - Fire extinguisher
   - Cell phone or change for public phone

3. Do you have the paperwork needed?
   - Record of pesticides carried (while no longer required by DOT, it's a good idea in case of an accident involving a spill)
   - Labels and MSDS's for pesticides carried
   - Pesticide emergency contacts & phone numbers

4. Are you taking precautions to prevent accidental poisoning?
   - No pesticides or sprayers stored in the cab
   - No lunches, other food, or cigarettes stored with pesticides
   - No children or pets riding where pesticides are stored
   - No oversupply of pesticides on board
   - Vehicle locked at all times

ELECTRIC SHOCK

Roughly one in ten workplace fatalities are caused by electrocutions. You face electrical hazards in a number of ways: damaged electrical tools, bad electrical grounds, spraying onto or drilling into live electrical lines, directly contacting live wires (such as in crawlspaces, attics, or in industrial accounts), indirectly contacting overhead wires with aluminum or other metal ladders, even from lightning strikes.

Electric shock occurs when the human body becomes part of an electric current. The electricity enters at one point, say your hand, is conducted through the body, and exits at another point, say your left foot. Injuries are varied and include direct effects such as burns, muscle and tendon damage, seizures, respiratory arrest, ventricular fibrillation (a deadly heart rhythm disturbance), and death. The extent of injuries depends on the size and duration of the current flow, electrical resistance, and the pathway through the body. Conduction from arm to arm or arm to foot is common in occupational accidents; it is also the most dangerous because the pathway leads through the heart. Even low voltage ranging 110-220 volts traveling through the heart for a fraction of a second can induce a dangerous and even deadly ventricular fibrillation. Indirect effects are also common; the person shocked may fall and injure himself, or let go of something and injure someone else.

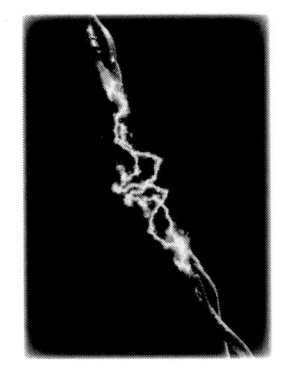

Ten percent of workplace fatalities are electrocutions

Photo © David Asch/iStockphoto

Grounded Equipment

Most industrial power tools are grounded through a third wire that runs from the casing to a grounding prong on the plug (see *Hand and Power Tools*). If the casing of the tool you are holding becomes energized because of a short, the ground is "the path of least resistance." It carries the current through the cord to the ground wires in the electrical system, and ultimately into a cold water pipe or a ground rod.

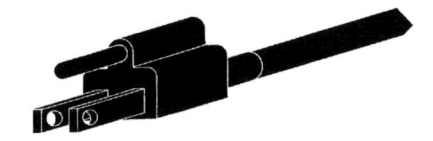

The grounding prong carries the electric current away from you if the tool you are holding becomes energized

But if the grounding prong is missing from the plug, or if the receptacle is ungrounded, your body becomes the path of least resistance. You can get a shock... perhaps a fatal one.

> *Precautions When Using Electric Tools*
> - Never remove a grounding prong or bypass the ground!
> - Use only grounded tools or double-insulated tools (double-insulated tools isolate the tool's outer case from the internal wiring).
> - Inspect all tools and cords prior to use.
> - Do not use a tool with a damaged cord or with a cracked outer case.
> - Use professional extension cords, fully grounded.
> - Be sure that plugs are completely inserted into receptacles.
> - If you feel a mild shock, stop using the tool and do not use it again until it is checked by a trained service person.
> - Report any electrical problems to your supervisor.
> - A receptacle circuit tester can check that the electrical path to the ground is continuous.
> - Use a ground fault interrupter (GFI) if you are working in a wet area.

Ground Fault Interrupter

Some pest control work sites present a higher than normal risk of electric shock because they are wet or damp and, therefore, highly conductive. Examples include a wet crawlspace or an industrial room with standing water. Double-insulated tools and grounded tools, which protect you from shock in normal situations, may not work in these wet sites. For example, you can be electrocuted if you drop an electric tool into water, or if you handle a frayed extension cord while standing in water and touching a conductive surface.

The Occupational Safety and Health Administration (OSHA) requires that portable electric equipment and flexible cords used in locations where employees are likely to contact water or conductive liquids be approved for those locations.

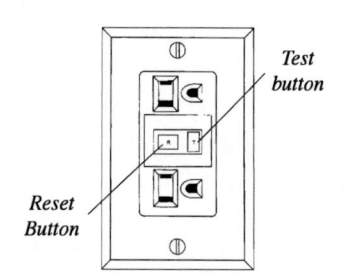

A receptacle-type ground fault interupter (GFI) protects you from shock in wet areas

But since neither double insulation nor grounding can guarantee protection in these sites, the use of a ground fault interrupter (GFI) is also necessary.

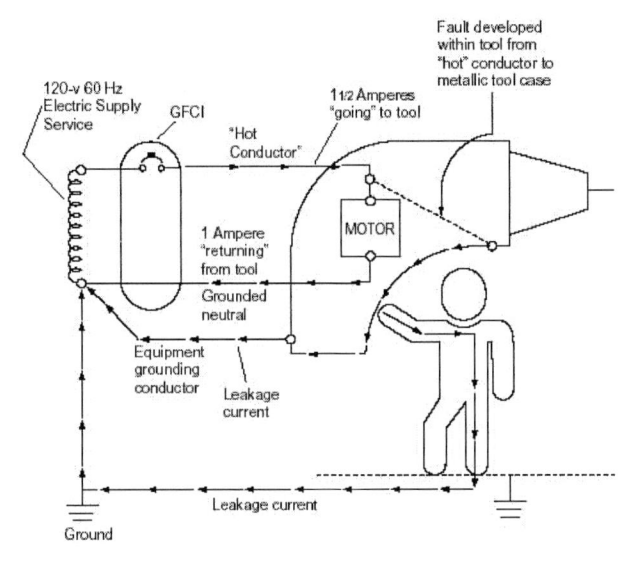

A GFI will open the circuit and cut off power in case of a short in the tool or wiring

    A ground fault interrupter (also called a ground fault circuit interrupter, or GFCI) is not a fuse or circuit breaker. It's a solid-state, specialized device that senses an imbalance in current flowing through a circuit. It can then open the circuit and cut off the power within a fortieth of a second, protecting the operator from serious shock. A GFI will open the circuit in case of ground fault leakage too small to trip the circuit breaker, but large enough to be dangerous to people.

    GFIs are of several types that can be placed at various points along the circuit-- in a panel box as a breaker, at the receptacle, or in line anywhere along an extension cord. It is best, however, not to place a GFI right at the tool. Instead, place it as far back towards the power receptacle as possible so that the extension cord, as well as the tool, is protected.

    Ground fault interrupters are not to be used instead of double-insulated tools or equipment grounding. GFIs are supplemental equipment used as a backup to normal precautions.

    Use a GFI with power tools whenever possible, and always when you are working in wet areas or drilling slabs with standing water. Also use a GFI whenever using high-pressure spray washers. Some of these washers are equipped with a GFI on the plug, some are not. Test portable GFIs before each use. GFIs have test and reset buttons to assure that the ground fault protection is still functioning.

> ### When GFIs Won't Protect You
>
> Be aware that GFIs are not 100% effective in preventing shocks. GFIs will not provide protection if, for some reason, you should contact the hot and the neutral wire while you are not grounded (line-to-line short). As the current through you is not flowing to ground, the GFI will not trigger.
>
> Also, GFIs will not protect you if you contact a different electrical circuit than the one the GFI is connected to. For example, if a saw or drill plugged into a GFI penetrates wiring of a circuit different than the one supplying its own power, you will not be protected from electrical shock unless the line you drill into also is protected by a GFI.

Protecting Yourself When Drilling Slabs

Whenever you drill through a slab you face some degree of risk of contacting a live electrical line. GFIs won't usually protect you from this risk (see box above). A "drill stop" may. It is an electronic device designed to stop power to a drill upon contact between the drill bit and grounded metal piping, electrical conduit, or reinforcement steel. (It is also equipped with one or more GFIs.)

Since a drill stop can help a drill operator avoid drilling through the grounded metal object, it may also prevent a shock caused by drilling into a live electrical line.

Be aware, though, that a drill stop only works if the conduit is properly installed and grounded. A drill stop, like a GFI, is not 100% effective.

Rubber gloves or heavy (and dry) leather gloves can insulate your body from your drill and so help protect you from electric shock from drilling into a live wire.

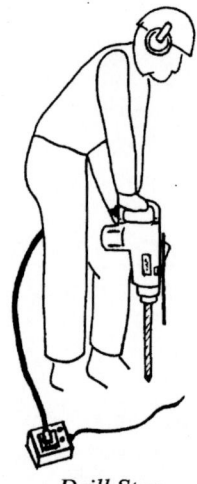

Drill Stop

A "drill stop" may prevent you from drilling into an electrical conduit

Connecting Plugs

Do not plug or unplug electrical tools or extension cords if either your hands or the plugs are wet. When using locking-type plugs, make sure that you completely lock them in.

Contacting Electrical Circuits During Application

Water conducts electricity, so you should not apply water-based pesticide near live electrical circuits. Application equipment may conduct electricity as well, so the tips of sprayers and dusters should be kept away from electrical receptacles and wiring. Dusters can be equipped with plastic or rubber tips that isolate you from any live electrical lines the tips might touch.

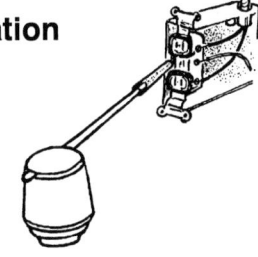

A plastic or rubber tip can prevent electric shock

Aluminum Ladders

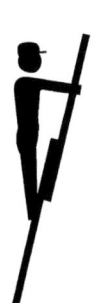

Roughly four percent of work-related electrocutions occur because portable aluminum ladders, which are electrical conductors, come in contact with energized overhead power lines. Here are basic rules regarding ladders and electric shock:

1. Do not use portable metal or conductive ladders for electrical work or where they may touch electrical conductors.
2. Tie, block, or otherwise secure an aluminum or other conductive ladder to prevent its falling or sliding onto an energized line that you do not know is nearby.

Overhead Power Lines

Many homes, apartments, and businesses are served by overhead power lines. Normally on the job, you're not in a position to even think about what's overhead. But there are times when you may find yourself up on a ladder or up on a roof using a bee pole, doing bird or bat control, trapping squirrels, removing wasp nests, inspecting roofs or chimneys, or installing vents.

You can be electrocuted or seriously injured by contact with an overhead power line if you do not take the proper precautions. You don't have to touch a power line directly to be electrocuted. You can be zapped just the same if you touch a conductive material (metal ladder, pruning pool, other tool) that is in contact with the line and, at the same time, touch the earth or a grounded item (metal siding, downspout).

- Before you approach the roof, check out the location of the power lines.
- Always assume that power lines are live. Even though there may be a weatherproofing covering on the line, that doesn't mean it's safe to touch. Many overhead power lines are not insulated.

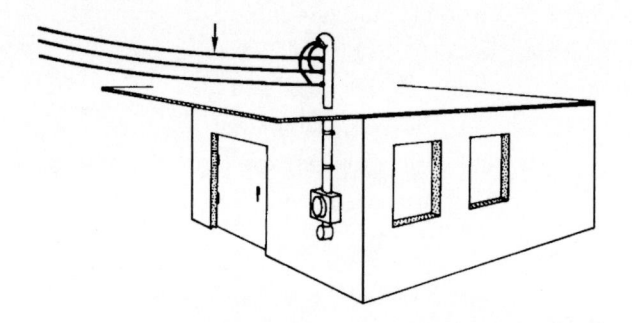

Look out for overhead power lines when working with ladders or using a bee pole

- Keep yourself, your ladder, and your equipment at least 10 feet away from power lines at all times.
- If working on a roof puts you close to overhead power lines, avoid standing up and accidentally touching a line with your head or shoulder.
- Consider your ladder material. Aluminum is an especially good conductor of electricity. People are also a natural conductor of electricity. Do not use an aluminum ladder where you know there are live exposed electrical conductors. Use a fiberglass or wooden ladder instead. In other areas, tie, block, or otherwise secure an aluminum or other conductive ladder to prevent it from falling or sliding onto an unrecognized energized line. (See previous section.)
- If cutting tree limbs that are overhanging the roof, note where the power lines are. If there is any chance that a limb could fall on a power line, contact the local power utility to de-energize and ground the line before you cut.
- If you are pruning tree limbs with a long-handled metal pruner, be very careful not to touch any power lines or any limbs that are touching power lines. Don't climb in trees that are near overhead power lines.

- Stay well away from a downed power line. You don't know whether it's a live line or not. Notify the local power utility.

Industrial Sites

Old manufacturing plants and other industrial sites may have unshielded wire or bare angle iron conductors carrying high voltage. Electrical cranes and hoist trolleys may be powered through open, exposed conductors. Such unshielded electrical conductors are always dangerous to a technician working near them on a ladder or man lift, or using pesticide application equipment. Even shielded conductors can be dangerous if they are not maintained properly and become cracked, frayed, or otherwise damaged. Stay alert to the risk of electrical shock when working in industrial sites, and learn to recognize potential electrical hazards.

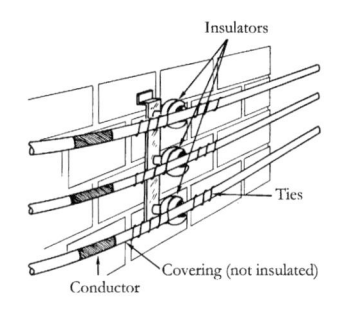

Watch out for unshielded wire and open conductors at industrial sites

Working Outside in Thunderstorms...Just Don't

Most lightning strikes occur from June through August. While death from lightning strikes in the U.S. is rare (about 70 deaths a year), nervous system damage is the most common injury. If you're working outside, as soon as you hear thunder, it's time to close up shop and take shelter. Lightning can travel 10 miles from the main rain area of a storm; that's about as far as you can hear thunder.

- The best place to be during a thunderstorm is indoors in a building that is grounded by wires and pipes. If you can't get inside, take shelter in your vehicle. Most people think that it is the rubber tires that protect you from lightning, but it's actually the metal shell of the vehicle that conducts the charge around you and into the ground.
- When you hear thunder, stop working with any power tools like hammer drills. [Likewise if you are inside during a lightning storm, you should not be working with power tools or anything plugged into a circuit.]
- Don't use any metal objects outside, electric or otherwise, if lightning is nearby. Metal objects don't attract lightning but they do conduct electricity. It's especially important to get away from aluminum ladders. Don't use any

kind of metal pole such as a catchpole or insect net. Stay away from metal fences.
- If you're working up high, like on a roof, get down immediately. Lightning strikes at the tallest object it can find. Fireplaces can conduct lightning too. Never take shelter under a tree since tall trees attract lightning, as do poles or towers.
- Stay away from any plumbing or pipes, whether outdoors or indoors. Do not use a hose or run water in a sink.
- Don't use a land phone line if there is thunder and lightning. Lightning can be conducted through the phone lines. It's okay to use cell phones.
- If you're working in or near water, get away. Holding a metal termiticide rod in a wet trench is not safe.
- The most dangerous time for a lightning strike is after you think the storm has passed. Don't be too quick to get back to work; there is often that one last boom and flash, even with blue sky overhead. More than half of all lightning deaths occur after the storm seems to have moved on.

Key Points to Remember—Electric Shock

- √ **Never remove a grounding prong or bypass the ground.**
- √ **Use only grounded tools or double-insulated tools (double-insulated tools isolate the tool's outer case from the internal wiring).**
- √ **Do not use equipment with damaged cords or cracked casings.**
- √ **If you feel a mild shock, stop using the tool.**
- √ **Use a ground fault interrupter (GFI) when drilling through a slab and when using any electrical tool in a wet area.**
- √ **Do not use portable metal or conductive ladders where they may contact electrical conductors.**
- √ **Do not apply water-based pesticide near live electrical circuits.**
- √ **Use a plastic or rubber tip on a metal duster spout.**
- √ **Before you place a ladder or use a bee pole, look overhead for power lines.**
- √ **Do not work outside during thunderstorms.**

ERGONOMICS AND MUSCULOSKELETAL DISORDERS

Ergonomics is the science of fitting jobs to the people who work in them. The goal of an ergonomics program is to reduce work-related musculoskeletal disorders (MSDs) developed by workers when a major part of their jobs involve reaching, bending over, lifting heavy objects, using continuous force, working with vibrating equipment and doing repetitive motions.

More than one hundred different types of job-induced injuries and illnesses are classified as musculoskeletal disorders, also called repetitive stress injuries (see box). They can occur any time there is a mismatch between the physical requirements of the job and the physical capacity of the human body.

Some Common Work-related Musculoskeletal Disorders (MSDs)

MSDs can affect muscles, nerves, tendons, ligaments, joints or spinal discs, and include the following conditions:

Carpal tunnel syndrome • Rotator cuff syndrome

De Quervain's disease • Trigger finger • Sciatica • Epicondylitis

Tendinitis • Raynaud's phenomenon • Carpet-layers' knee

Herniated spinal disc • Low back pain

Hand-arm vibration syndrome (HAVS) • Tension neck syndrome

Workplace MSDs are caused by exposure to one or more of the following five risk factors:

1. **Repetition.** Doing the same motions over and over places stress on the muscles and tendons. The severity of risk depends on how often the action is repeated, the speed of the movement, the number of muscles involved and the required force.
2. **Forceful Exertions.** Force is the amount of physical effort required to perform a task (such as heavy lifting) or to maintain control of equipment or tools. The amount of force depends on the type of grip, the weight of an object, body posture, the type of activity and the duration of the task.
3. **Awkward Postures.** Posture is the position your body is in and affects muscle groups that are involved in physical activity. Awkward postures include repeated or prolonged reaching, twisting, bending, kneeling, squatting, working overhead with your hands or arms, or holding fixed positions.

4. **Contact Stress.** Pressing the body repeatedly against a hard or sharp edge can result in placing too much pressure on nerves, tendons and blood vessels. For example, using the palm of your hand as a hammer can increase your risk of suffering an MSD.
5. **Vibration.** Operating vibrating tools such as hammer drills, sanders, grinders, chippers, routers, and saws can lead to nerve damage (See *Hand-Arm Vibration Syndrome*, later in this section.

Signs and Symptoms of Musculoskeletal Disorders

Workers suffering from MSDs may experience less strength for gripping, less range of motion, loss of muscle function and inability to do everyday tasks. Common symptoms include the following:

Painful joints • Pain in wrists, shoulders, forearms, knees • Stiffness

Pain, tingling or numbness in hands or feet • Back or neck pain

Fingers or toes turning white (blanching) • Burning sensations

Shooting or stabbing pains in arms or legs • Swelling or inflammation

Risk of Musculoskeletal Disorders in Pest Control

The highest risk of MSDs is probably from computer data entry by office staff, which can cause carpal tunnel syndrome to the hands and arms. This syndrome occurs when a certain ligament in your arm becomes inflamed and compresses a nerve that runs to the fingers. Constant text messaging may cause a similar problem. Symptoms include pain in the arm and numbness and tingling in the hands and fingers. Untreated, it may lead to severely disabling muscle weakness in the hands. Carpal tunnel syndrome causes more days off work than any other injury!

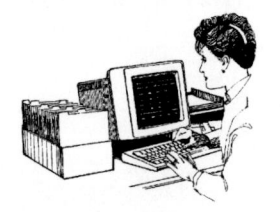

Carpal tunnel syndrome causes more lost work days than any other injury

A pest control technician's job is usually so varied that a work-related MSD is not likely. An exception might be if you are performing the same task, day after day, week after week, such as drilling holes in concrete or loading/unloading in the warehouse. Hammer drills, for example, can cause <u>h</u>and-<u>a</u>rm <u>v</u>ibration <u>s</u>yndrome, or HAVS for short, which is discussed below.

If you suspect you may be developing a MSD, contact your supervisor right away. It is important to identify such injury early to prevent serious illness, injury, or disability. A simple change in procedure or equipment is often all that is necessary.

Hand-Arm Vibration Syndrome

Vibrating hand tools, such as hammer drills used in termite work and chain saws, can cause an uncommon medical condition called hand-arm vibration syndrome, or HAVS for short. Other names include vibration white finger, dead hand, and Raynaud's phenomenon. The signs and symptoms of HAVS include tingling or numbness, pain, and blanching (the fingers, starting at the tips, turning pale and ashen) caused by reduced blood circulation. Early symptoms occur most often early in the morning, driving to work (hands on a cold steering wheel), and when hands are cold and wet. Attacks typically last 15-60 minutes, but in advanced cases may last up to two hours. With continuing exposure to vibration, the signs and symptoms become more severe and frequent, making it difficult to pick up small objects, zipper or button clothing, etc. The condition may eventually become irreversible with a narrowing of blood vessels in the fingers. Serious symptoms can begin occurring after as little as one year's exposure to vibration.

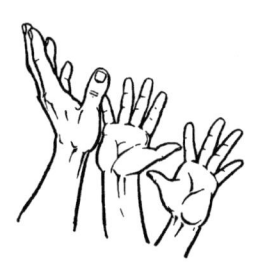

Vibrating tools can affect circulation

Precautions to Avoid HAVS

- When using a hammer drill, chain saw, or a similar vibrating tool, let the tool do the work. Don't force it. Pressure increases the vibration that is passed to the hands.
- Schedule a ten-minute break every hour when using a hammer drill or other vibrating hand tool.
- Make sure vibrating hand tools are maintained according to manufacturer's specifications (out of adjustment, dull, or poorly maintained tools can vibrate excessively).
- In cold or wet weather, wear adequate clothing and keep hands warm and dry (cold can trigger a HAVS attack). More than one pair of gloves may be required to keep

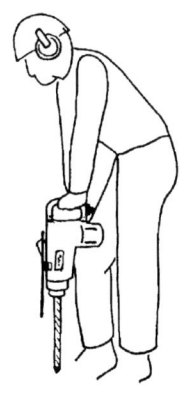

Don't force it. Let the tool do the work

hands warm and reduce vibration. Special anti-vibration gloves are also available.
- Do not smoke when using vibrating hand tools since smoking restricts blood circulation to hands and arms.
- Tell your supervisor if you have lasting symptoms of tingling or numbness (temporary tingling or numbness right after using a tool is not a symptom of HAVS), or signs of blanched or blue fingers. See a physician.

Key Points to Remember—Ergonomics and MSDs

- √ *Workplace musculoskeletal disorders are caused by exposure to repetition, forceful exertions, awkward postures, contact stress, or vibration.*
- √ *Workers suffering from musculoskeletal disorders may experience less strength for gripping, less range of motion, loss of muscle function, and inability to do everyday tasks.*
- √ *If you suspect you may be developing repetitive stress injury, contact your supervisor.*
- √ *A simple change in procedure will often prevent repetitive stress injury.*
- √ *Vibrating hand tools can cause an uncommon medical condition called hand-arm vibration syndrome, or HAVS for short.*
- √ *Symptoms of HAVS include tingling or numbness, pain, and blanching of the fingers, starting at the tips.*
- √ *When using a hammer drill or similar tool, let the tool do the work.*
- √ *Schedule a ten-minute break every hour when using a hammer drill or other vibrating hand tool.*

FIBERGLASS INSULATION

Do you ever work in attics or other sites containing insulation? Then you need to know about the potential health risk of fiberglass and mineral wool insulation.

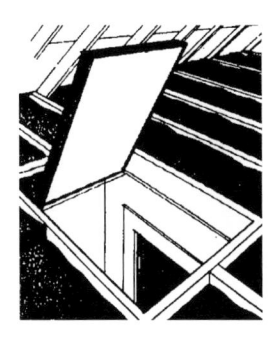

These materials are commonly used for "blown-in" insulation (although cellulose is an alternative) and in batts (sheets) of insulation covered on one side with brown Kraft paper.

The MSDSs for such products now have warning statements such as, *"Fiberglass wool is a possible cancer hazard by inhalation and may cause irritation of upper respiratory tract. Use of a respirator such as 3M model 9900 or equivalent is recommended."* There are also warnings of "mechanical irritations" of the skin, eyes, and upper respiratory tract. These warnings are mainly aimed at installers but also apply to anyone working around these materials.

Be careful of fiberglass when inspecting or treating attics

There are three ways you might be exposed to fiberglass: (1) by breathing airborne fibers after you have disturbed the insulation, (2) through direct skin contact (touching or crawling over the insulation), and (3) through indirect contact (transferring fibers from your clothes to your skin or eyes, or even by passing fibers to other clothes in the laundry). Your highest exposure would likely occur when inspecting or treating an attic with blown-in insulation.

Precautions When Working Around Insulation

- Disturb insulation as little as possible, particularly blown-in and/or loose insulation in an attic.
- Wear a respirator if there is a risk of airborne fibers, such as when you move insulation while inspecting for pests, or when using a power duster.
- Wear long sleeves and pants (loose fitting) and gloves (cotton is OK).
- Wear Tyvek® or similar coveralls, head covering (cap, hat, or hood), and safety goggles if you must work directly in or on the insulation, or if

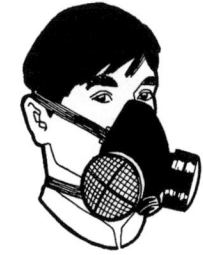

The proper respirator will filter fiberglass particles

you have experienced irritation or sensitivity to fiberglass insulation in the past.
- If you experience skin or eye irritation, or coughing or other evidence of respiratory exposure, leave the area and reassess safety procedures.
- In case of eye irritation or contact, flush eyes with clean water for 15 minutes.
- Do not wear contact lenses.
- Brush off clothing before entering your vehicle.
- Wash exposed skin with soap and water. Shower after work. Use skin cream to soothe irritation. If skin, eye, or lung irritation persists, consult a physician.
- Wash contaminated clothing separately, and rinse the washer afterwards.

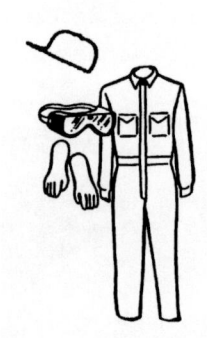

PPE that can protect you from direct skin contact with fiberglass

Key Points to Remember—Fiberglass Insulation

- √ **Fiberglass insulation is a possible cancer hazard by inhalation and may cause irritation of the skin, eyes, and upper respiratory tract by contact.**
- √ **There are three ways you might be exposed: (1) by breathing airborne fibers, (2) through direct skin contact, and (3) through indirect contact (for example, transferring fibers from clothes to skin or eyes).**
- √ **A technician's greatest risk of exposure is inspecting or treating an attic with blown-in fiberglass insulation.**
- √ **Disturb insulation as little as possible, particularly blown-in and/or loose insulation in an attic.**
- √ **Wear a respirator when you disturb insulation or when using a power duster.**
- √ **Wear coveralls, head covering, and safety goggles if you must work directly in or on the insulation, or if you know you are sensitive to it.**

FIRE

The first consideration when a fire is discovered is not putting out the fire, but how to best protect yourself and others from injury.

Fire Emergency Procedures

If You Discover a Fire in a Building:
1. Activate the nearest fire alarm.
2. Notify the fire department or dial 911. Give your location, the nature of the fire, and your name.

Fight the Fire ONLY if:
1. The fire department has been notified of the fire, AND
2. The fire is small and confined to its area of origin, AND
3. You have a way out and can fight the fire with your back to the exit, AND
4. You have the proper extinguisher, in good working order, AND know how to use it, AND
5. Pesticides are not burning or are not about to burn.
6. If you are not sure of your ability or the fire extinguisher's capacity to contain the fire, *or if pesticides are involved*, leave the area.

If You Hear a Fire Alarm:
1. Evacuate the area. Close windows, turn off any gas jets, and close doors as you leave.
2. Leave the building and move away from exits and out of the way of emergency operations. Do not use elevators.
3. Assemble in a designated area.
4. Report to a fire monitor or other official so he can determine that all personnel have evacuated your area.
5. Remain outside until a competent authority states that it is safe to re-enter.

Leave the building if you hear a fire alarm; don't use elevators

In Case of a Vehicle Fire:
1. Get out of your vehicle.
2. Grab your respirator and fire extinguisher if possible.

3. If the fire is small and confined to its area of origin, fight the fire.
4. Wear your respirator if the fire is burning near pesticides.
5. If you are not sure of your ability or the fire extinguisher's capacity to contain the fire, *or if pesticides are involved,* get away from the vehicle and move people away.
6. Notify the fire department or dial 911. Give your location, the nature of the fire, the fact that the vehicle contains pesticides, and your name.

Fires Involving Pesticides

A fire where pesticides are stored (either in a building or in your vehicle) can be extremely dangerous. Besides the simple fact that there's a fire that can destroy property and threaten life, a pesticide fire can release toxic smoke and fumes that can affect people over a wide area. Some pesticides act as oxidizers, fueling extremely hot fires that quickly flare out of control. Pesticides containing oil or petroleum-based solvents have the lowest flash points, and therefore usually ignite more easily.

Your first concern in a fire is protecting yourself and others. If you detect a fire in an area where pesticides or other chemicals are stored:

- Activate the nearest fire alarm.
- Notify a supervisor if one is immediately available. If not, notify the fire department or dial 911. Give your location and your name and be sure to alert officials that the fire is in a chemical storage area. If you can, identify the types of pesticides or chemicals involved.

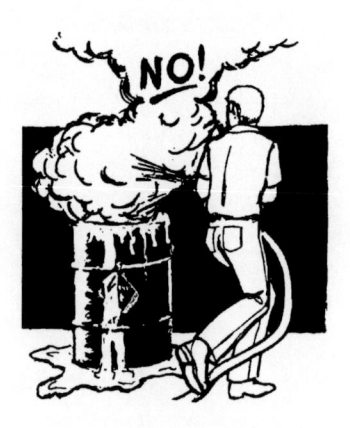

Never attempt to fight a pesticide fire

Fire Extinguishers

Fire extinguishers are classified for different types of fires. Extinguishers that are approved for use on burning wood (Class **A**) may not be adequate to fight a chemical fire (Class **B**) or an electrical fire (Class **C**). Many *dry chemical* extinguishers are multipurpose and are labeled for **A-B-C** fires. All extinguishers are labeled with one or more picture or letter symbols that give the class of extinguisher and type of fire it can handle.

If a fire is small when discovered, you can probably put it out with a fire extinguisher...but act fast, and consider your own safety first. Stay near an escape door. Don't let yourself get trapped. If the fire is already large, don't try to fight it. Get out and get help.

- Be familiar with the use directions on the fire extinguisher. Most simply require that you pull out the lock pin, aim at the base of the fire, and squeeze the handle.
- When using a *dry chemical* extinguisher for any type of fire (A, B, or C), coat the burning surface with chemical using a side-to-side motion. This procedure is sometimes abbreviated as PASS: Pull, Aim, Squeeze, Sweep.

PASS! *Pull, Aim, Squeeze, Sweep*

A fire extinguisher seems like a fairly obvious piece of equipment. But if you've never actually had the occasion to use one, you could draw a blank when the time comes. There's an acronym that can help you...PASS. PASS stands for Pull, Aim, Squeeze, Sweep.

PULL -- You can't begin to do anything with a fire extinguisher unless you first pull the pin that locks the handle.

AIM - This one isn't as simple as it sounds. You have to aim at the base of the fire. If you aim at the flames (which is the natural tendency), the discharge will pass right through and do no good.

SQUEEZE - Once you've removed the pin and pointed the fire extinguisher at the base of the fire, then squeeze the top handle to release the discharge.

SWEEP - Slowly sweep from side to side across the base of the burning area until the fire is completely out. Stand back at a safe distance while sweeping and gradually move forward as you control the fire. When using a foam type fire extinguisher, don't splash the foam onto the fire. Curve the foam discharge up slightly so that it falls lightly, or aim it behind the fire at a wall and let it flow onto the fire. Cover all surfaces with foam.

Note: Once the fire is out, have someone keep an eye on it in case it reignites.

- When using a *foam* type fire extinguisher for combustible liquid (class B) or electrical equipment (class C) fires, curve the foam discharge up slightly so that it falls lightly, or aim it behind the fire at a wall and let it flow onto the fire. Cover all surfaces with foam.
- Even after a fire appears to be out, stand by in case the fire rekindles.
- When fighting an electrical (class C) fire, shut off the main electrical supply switch at the breaker box as soon as possible.
- When fighting a fire of burning pesticides or other chemicals...**don't!** These fires can produce deadly smoke or fumes. Don't try to extinguish burning chemicals. Anyone fighting such a fire must wear special protective gear, including an air-supplied respirator. Evacuate the area and call the fire department.

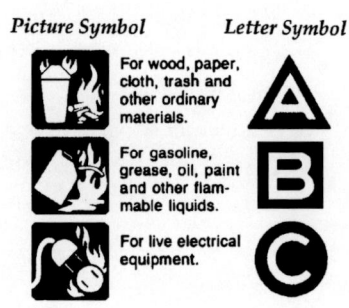

Picture Symbol		Letter Symbol
	For wood, paper, cloth, trash and other ordinary materials.	A
	For gasoline, grease, oil, paint and other flammable liquids.	B
	For live electrical equipment.	C

Extinguishers are labeled for their approved uses

Pesticide Flash Point

Flash point is the lowest temperature at which a combustible liquid will give off a flammable vapor. In other words, the temperature at which a pesticide will ignite. You'll find this information on the material safety data sheet (MSDS) under a heading like "Fire and Explosion Hazard Data." It may say, "Flash point: 94° F." or "Flash point: over 200° F." or "Flash point: Not applicable." Pesticides containing oil or petroleum-based solvents usually ignite more easily and, therefore, have the lowest flash points.

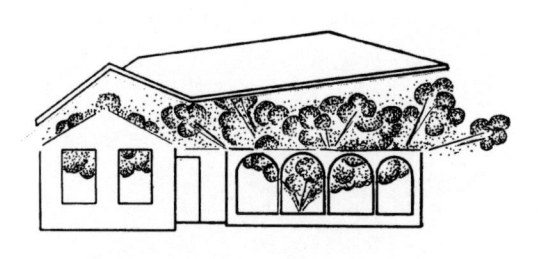

Overdosed flammable aerosols and flames don't mix!

Do you need to be concerned about the flash point of the chemicals you use? Yes. A pesticide at a temperature above its flash point is giving off a vapor that could ignite (and, of course, that vapor is toxic, too). Pesticides with low flash points must be protected from flame, direct sunlight, and heat sources...even a hot vehicle interior on a summer day.

If you do space treatments around open flames with products having a low flash point, you risk fire or explosion. The more chemical you apply, the greater the risk that the vapors will reach their explosive limit. You've probably read newspaper stories about homeowners who have set off 20 aerosol "bombs" at one time, thinking that more was better. They forgot to turn off the pilot lights, they overdosed the area with vapors, and...KABOOM!

If you're doing a space treatment, check the product label and the MSDS flash point information. Don't overdose, because higher concentrations may have higher risks of ignition. When treating with a flammable product around stoves, water heaters, or space heaters--anything that is extremely hot or has an open flame--turn it off and extinguish the flame first. If you ignore this advice and you see the flame on the stove or water heater start to brighten, you're about to get a real hands-on demonstration of the meaning of the term "flash point."

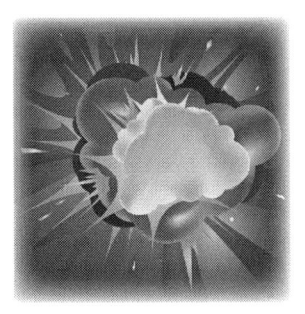

Do not get a hands-on demonstration of the term "flash-point"!

Graphic © susaro/iStockphoto

When NOT to Fight a Fire

Do not attempt to fight the fire unless (1) the fire department has been notified, (2) the fire is small and confined, (3) you have a way out and can fight the fire with your back to the exit (don't let yourself be trapped!), (4) you have the proper extinguisher, in good working order, and know how to use it, and (5) *pesticides are not directly involved in the fire.*

If you are not sure of any one of these five items, do not attempt to fight the fire. Once again, never attempt to fight a fire if the fire involves or is about to involve pesticides or other chemicals. This is a job for specially trained firefighters with special protective gear, including air-supplied respirators. Even the water used to fight a pesticide fire has to be contained or specially handled to prevent run-off contamination of streams and property.

Your company may prohibit attempting to fight a fire under any circumstances. Check with your supervisor regarding company policy.

Pest Control Technician Safety Manual

Key Points to Remember—Fire

- √ *Your first concern in a fire is protecting yourself and others.*
- √ *If you are not sure of your ability to fight a fire, move yourself and others away.*
- √ *Don't try to extinguish burning chemicals. Evacuate the area and call the fire department.*
- √ *When using a dry chemical extinguisher, PASS: Pull, Aim, Squeeze, Sweep the burning surface.*
- √ *When using a foam type fire extinguisher, curve the foam discharge up slightly so that it falls lightly.*
- √ *When space-treating (fogging) around a stove, water heater, or space heater--anything that is extremely hot or has an open flame--turn it off and extinguish the flame first.*

FIREARMS

We don't generally think of firearms as a pest control tool. Yet in some parts of the country, pest control technicians may use rifles, shotguns, or airguns to control nuisance birds, snakes, squirrels, and other wildlife. The safety issue, of course, is what the military likes to call "collateral damage," meaning the risk that something or someone accidently stops a bullet.

If you use any type of firearm, follow state regulations and these rules:

- Always keep the muzzle pointed in a safe direction.
- Treat every firearm as though it were loaded.
- Always make sure the firearm is unloaded and keep the action open except when preparing to shoot.
- Be sure the barrel and action are clear of obstruction and that you have the proper ammunition for the firearm you are carrying.
- Be sure of your target before you pull the trigger.
- Never point a firearm at anything you do not want to shoot.
- Do not engage in horseplay with any firearm.
- Never climb a ladder, fence, tree, or jump a ditch carrying a loaded firearm.
- Never shoot at a flat hard surface or water.

- Store firearms and ammunition separately.
- When carrying firearms in a vehicle, keep them unloaded, locked in a case, and have your ammunition locked and stored separately.
- Prevent unauthorized access to firearms.
- Avoid alcohol and other drugs before or during shooting.
- Wear ear protection and safety glasses.

Airguns

Airguns are not toys. They are very effective at killing birds and small animals, and are sometimes used for pest control. Serious airguns (not BB guns) shoot pellets (bullets) ranging from .177 to .25 caliber at muzzle velocities of 1,000 fps or more...powerful enough to kill a raccoon.

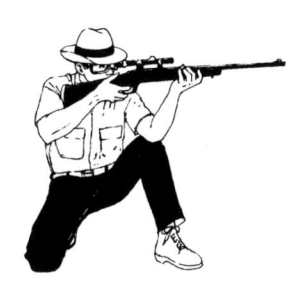

Airguns are powerful and effective killing tools

When using an airgun, use the proper pressure. To kill a squirrel, pigeon, or starling requires about 3 ft-lbs at the point of impact. Since a fully pumped airgun will typically provide 10-25 ft-lbs of energy at 10 yards, you don't need to fully pump for every shot. Two or three pumps will typically be sufficient, and reduce the risk of ricochet and collateral damage in case of a miss. Each pump increases the energy by roughly 10-15 percent.

Follow good safety practices with airguns just as you would with a regular firearm. Wear safety glasses. Do not shoot toward others (pellets can travel 500 yards or more, and can cause serious eye damage). Do not shoot where pellets could cause contamination or problems (food processing areas, over open mechanical equipment). Use a scope for accuracy.

Key Points to Remember—Firearms

- √ **Always keep the muzzle pointed in a safe direction.**
- √ **Treat every firearm as though it were loaded.**
- √ **Never point a firearm at anything you do not want to shoot.**
- √ **When not in use, keep firearms unloaded, locked in a case, and have your ammunition locked and stored separately.**
- √ **Follow good safety practices with airguns just as you would with a regular firearm.**

FIRST AID

You may face a situation where you need to apply first aid—to yourself, a coworker, a customer, or even a stranger. The injury could be as minor as a cut or as major as electric shock, or anything from an insect sting to a heart attack. Become familiar with first aid procedures. Make sure the first aid kit in your vehicle is where you can find it, and that it is fully stocked.

A good set of supplies for a basic first aid kit suitable for a pest control vehicle would include:

- gauze pads (at least 4 X 4 inches)
- two larger gauze pads (at least 8 X 10 inches)
- box of assorted Band-Aids®
- one package gauze roller bandage at least 2 inches wide
- two triangular bandages
- wound cleaning agent such as sealed moistened towelettes
- scissors
- at least one blanket
- tweezers
- adhesive tape
- latex gloves
- resuscitation equipment such as resuscitation bag, airway, or mouth mask
- two elastic wraps
- splint
- directions for requesting emergency assistance
- eye wash dispenser
- detergent and water
- milk of magnesia, activated charcoal and instructions on how to administer them in case of pesticide poisoning and when called for by the label

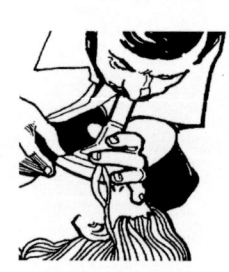

Use a mouth mask when doing CPR

To protect yourself from bloodborne pathogens when giving first aid, avoid contact with blood, wear gloves, and use a mouth mask if performing CPR (cardiopulmonary resuscitation).

See *Pesticide Poisoning* and *Stinging and Venomous Pests* for specific first aid recommendations for those situations.

Recommendations Related to CPR

The American Heart Association now recommends that anyone finding an unconscious person *immediately* call an ambulance.

Standard CPR procedure used to be to check breathing and pulse, and sometimes to administer CPR, before leaving the victim to call for help. But research has shown that about 80 percent of adults found unconscious are in ventricular fibrillation (VF), a life-threatening heart arrhythmia. CPR does not convert VF rhythm back to normal. Paramedics use a *defibrillator* to shock the heart back into regular rhythm...and the sooner the procedure starts, the more likelihood there is of success.

The American Heart Association decided that anything that could be done to speed the rescue team to the victim would improve the victim's chances, and thus the switch in emphasis -- *call an ambulance as soon as it is clear that a person is unconscious.* This policy applies only to unconscious victims older than 8 years old. Younger victims are more likely to suffer from choking or other respiratory arrest, which is better served by immediate CPR.

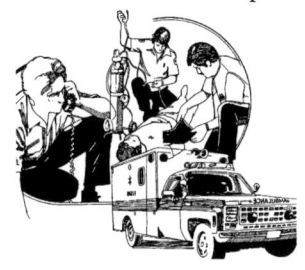

Immediately call an ambulance if someone is unconscious

Furthermore, the heart association has revised its CPR guidelines based on data collected from randomized trials of different rescue techniques. The most important finding of these trials is that the current recommendation to check for a pulse before beginning CPR increases the risk of death. Instead, the heart association recommends calling 911 and then starting CPR immediately, without bothering to check the pulse, if the victim is not breathing or moving. The sooner CPR is begun, the greater the chance of success.

Recognizing a Heart Attack

Not all chest pain means a heart attack. But nothing will get you to the front of the emergency room line faster than saying. "I am having chest pain." The risks are simply too great to ignore chest pain, whether yours or someone else's.

The start of a typical heart attack feels like pressure and a dull ache just under the sternum. People often describe it as a weight pressing on their chest. The ache and pressure can radiate down the left arm or into the neck, jaw, or stomach. Many people feel

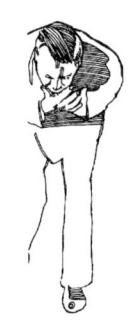

Never ignore chest pain

nauseous. The pain lasts longer than three minutes, and is usually not stabbing or sharp. But there are no absolutes. The pain may radiate down the right arm, or be felt somewhere else. People over 70, women, and diabetics may exhibit different symptoms.

The differences between the typical symptoms of a heart attack and noncardiac chest pain are shown below (but remember that symptoms can vary out of the normal). Whenever someone is experiencing chest pain that might signal a heart attack, get medical help immediately.

Symptoms: Heart Attack
- pressure and ache under sternum
- radiates to arm(s), neck
- lasts more than 3 minutes
- does not get worse after movement or breathing
- not affected by pressing on the chest
- not relieved by antacids

Symptoms: Noncardiac Chest Pain
- sharp,stabbing pain
- localized, does not radiate
- short-lived, usually less than 30 seconds
- gets worse after movement or breathing
- gets worse when chest is pressed
- relieved by antacids

Points to Remember — First Aid

- √ **Make sure the first aid kit in your vehicle is where you can find it, and that it is fully stocked.**
- √ **When giving first aid, avoid contact with blood, wear gloves, and use a mouth mask if performing CPR.**
- √ **If you find an unconscious person, you should immediately call an ambulance.**
- √ **Whenever someone is experiencing chest pain that might signal a heart attack, get medical help immediately.**

FLASHLIGHTS

You probably think of your flashlight as one of the safest pieces of equipment that you handle on a day-to-day basis. But the National Institute of Occupational Safety and Health (NIOSH) warns that there have been cases where flashlights have exploded on the job, injuring workers.

It's the batteries. Zinc/carbon and alkaline batteries naturally give off hydrogen gas. Differences in batteries and in the way that they're used affects the amount of gas that is given off.

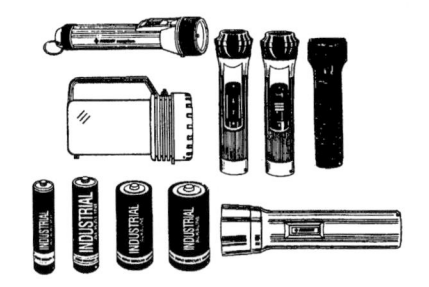

Periodically check the batteries in all of your flashlights for corrosion and leakage

Batteries and battery compartments usually allow the gradual release of any accumulated hydrogen gas. But some battery compartments, such as in waterproof flashlights, may be sealed tight against air and water by design. Although most of these flashlights have a pressure relief valve or use chemicals that absorb hydrogen gas, these safeguards many not be enough if batteries are used incorrectly.

Besides the potential for injury from flying parts, an exploding flashlight can release caustic chemicals and could start a fire or larger explosion in a flammable atmosphere.

Excess hydrogen gas is more likely to be released if you:

- mix different brands of batteries
- mix alkaline batteries with nonalkaline batteries
- mix old batteries with new batteries
- use damaged batteries
- insert the batteries incorrectly so that the polarity is reversed

Periodically check the batteries in your flashlight to make sure they're in good shape and not corroded. Opening the battery compartment will also allow any accumulated hydrogen gas to escape. But do not open your flashlight in a hazardous area or near an open flame.

Heat from Halogen Bulbs

Halogen and certain other flashlight bulbs may put out enough heat to cause a burn or ignite flammable materials if held in direct contact for a long period. A halogen flashlight left on in a back pocket can burn you if you sit on it, or melt the vinyl on the seat.

Key Points to Remember—Flashlights

- √ **Flashlights, particularly waterproof ones, have exploded on the job, injuring workers.**
- √ **Periodically check the batteries in your flashlight to make sure they're in good shape and not corroded.**
- √ **Do not open your flashlight in a hazardous area or near an open flame.**
- √ **Halogen bulbs put out enough heat to cause a burn.**

HAND AND POWER TOOLS

Tools are such a common part of our lives that we forget that they may pose hazards. Six basic safety rules can help you prevent injury when you use hand and power tools:

(1) Keep all tools in good condition with regular maintenance.
(2) Use the right tool for the job.
(3) Examine each tool for damage before use and do not use damaged tools.
(4) Operate tools according to the manufacturers' instructions.
(5) Use personal protective equipment when necessary.
(6) Store tools so as to avoid damage to the tools and cut and stick injuries to you or others.

If you encounter a hazardous situation with a tool that you cannot deal with on your own, bring it immediately to the attention of your supervisor.

Hand Tools

Hand tools are tools that are powered manually. They can include anything from axes to wrenches. The main hazards posed by hand tools are from improper use and improper maintenance. For example, if a wooden handle on a tool is loose or cracked, the head of the tool could fly off, striking the user or a bystander. Or, if an impact tool like a chisel, wedge, or drift pin has a mushroomed head, the head could shatter on impact, sending sharp fragments flying.

Safe tool handling is mostly common sense, tool maintenance, and paying attention to what you're doing.

- Wear appropriate personal protective equipment for the job such as safety goggles and gloves.
- Choose the right tool for the job and examine each tool before use.
- Don't use a wrench if the jaws are sprung to the point that slippage occurs.
- Direct the motion of saw blades, knives, and other tools away from people.
- Keep tools sharp. Dull tools are more hazardous than sharp ones.
- Avoid "mushrooming" the heads of impact tools like wedges or chisels.
- Iron or steel hand tools can produce sparks that can ignite flammables. When working where highly volatile liquids, flammable gases, or other potential explosives are stored, use spark-resistant tools.

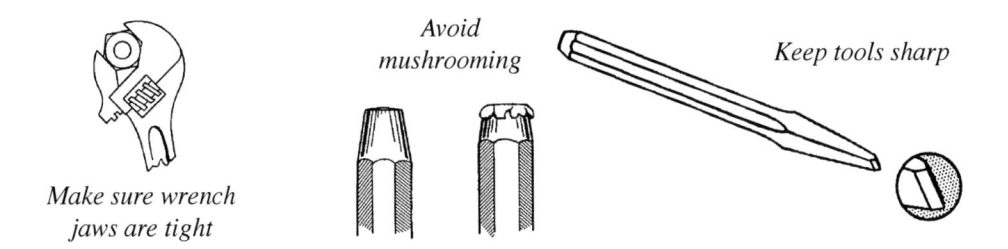

Make sure wrench jaws are tight

Avoid mushrooming

Keep tools sharp

Good tool maintenance not only keeps hand tools working efficiently, it helps you avoid accident and injury

If you question the safety of a tool or encounter a hazardous situation with a tool that you can't deal with on your own, bring it to the attention of your supervisor.

Power Tools

Power tools are classified by their power source: electric, pneumatic, liquid fuel, hydraulic, etc. To avoid accidents when using power tools, observe the following general precautions:

- Never carry a tool by the cord or hose.

Pest Control Technician Safety Manual

- Never yank the cord or the hose to disconnect it from the receptacle.
- Keep cords and hoses away from heat, oil, and sharp edges.
- Disconnect tools when not using them, before servicing and cleaning them, and when changing accessories such as blades, bits, and cutters.
- Keep all people not involved with the work at a safe distance from the work area.
- Secure work with clamps or a vise, freeing both hands to operate the tool.
- Avoid accidental starting. Do not hold fingers on the switch button while carrying a plugged-in tool.
- Maintain tools with care; keep them sharp and clean for best performance.
- Follow instructions in the user's manual for lubricating and changing accessories.
- Be sure to keep good footing and maintain good balance when operating power tools.
- Wear proper apparel for the task. Loose clothing, ties, or jewelry can catch in moving parts.
- Remove all damaged portable electric tools from use and tag them: "Do Not Use."

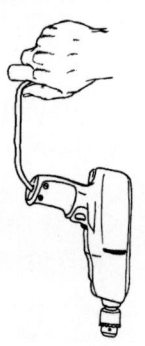

Never carry a tool by its cord or its hose

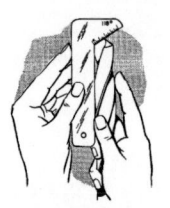

Keep bits and tools sharp

Guards

Belts, gears, shafts, pulleys, sprockets, spindles, drums, flywheels, chains, or other reciprocating, rotating, or moving parts of equipment must be guarded to protect you from injury, as must parts that throw off flying chips and sparks. Do not remove or bypass safety guards.

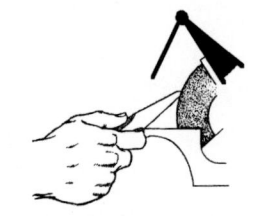

Use safety guards and don't remove them

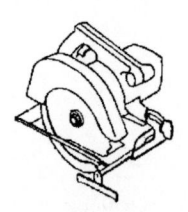

Portable circular saws having a blade greater than 2 inches (5.08 centimeters) in diameter must be equipped at all times with guards. An upper guard must cover the entire blade of the saw. A retractable lower guard must cover the teeth of the saw, except where it makes contact with the work material. The lower guard must automatically return to the covering position when the tool is withdrawn from the work material.

Circular saws must have upper and lower guards

Electric Tools

You face several hazards when using electric tools. Among the most serious are electrical burns and shocks. An electric shock also can cause the user to fall off of a ladder or other elevated work surface and be injured.

Electric tools must (1) have a three-wire cord with ground and be plugged into a grounded receptacle, (2) be double-insulated, or (3) be powered by a low-voltage isolation transformer. Three-wire cords contain two current-carrying conductors and a grounding conductor. Any time an adapter is used to accommodate a two-hole receptacle, the adapter wire must be attached to a known ground. *The third prong must never be removed from the plug.* If the grounding prong is missing, and the tool shorts-out and charges the outer case, you could be electrocuted.

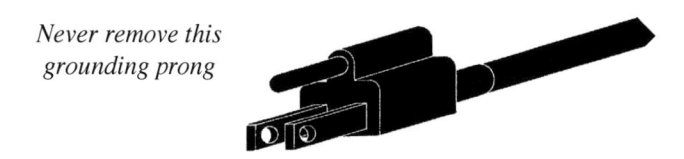

Never remove this grounding prong

Three-wire cords contain two current-carrying conductors and a grounding conductor.

Electric shock dangers from power tools and other sources are discussed in detail in the section titled *Electric Shock*. But in general, follow these rules when working with electric tools:

- Never carry a tool by the cord.
- Never yank the cord to disconnect it from the receptacle.
- Operate electric tools within their design limitations.
- Use gloves, eye protection, and appropriate safety footwear when using electric tools.
- Store electric tools in a dry place when not in use.
- Do not use electric tools in damp or wet locations unless they are approved for that purpose.
- Keep work areas well lighted when operating electric tools.

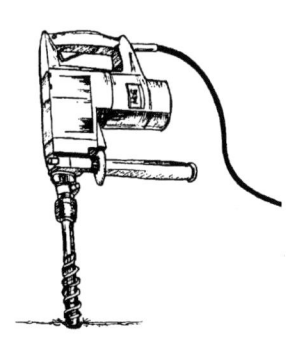

Be ready for the powerful torque of a large drill

- Ensure that cords from electric tools do not present a tripping hazard.
- When working in wet areas, plug electric tools into a GFI (ground fault interrupter) that is itself plugged into a grounded circuit (see *Electric Shock*).
- When drilling slabs, plug your drill or hammer-drill into a GFI.
- When using a high-torque drill, position yourself so that if the bit becomes stuck your hands or your body won't be smashed or pinned against a wall.

Pneumatic Tools

Pneumatic tools are powered by compressed air and include chippers, drills, hammers, and sanders. Follow these rules to minimize risks:

- Check pneumatic tools before each use and make sure the tool is fastened securely to the air hose to prevent it from becoming disconnected. Make sure there is a short wire or positive locking device attaching the air hose to the tool as an added safeguard.
- If an air hose is more than $^1/_2$ inch (12.7 millimeters) in diameter, a safety excess flow valve must be installed at the source of the air supply to reduce pressure in case of hose failure.
- In general, take the same precautions with an air hose as you would with electric cords, because the hose is subject to the same kind of damage or accidental striking, and because it also presents tripping hazards.

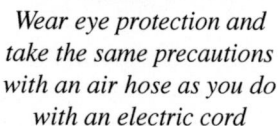

Wear eye protection and take the same precautions with an air hose as you do with an electric cord

- When using pneumatic tools, make sure that there is a safety clip or retainer installed to prevent attachments, such as chisels on a chipping hammer, from being ejected during tool operation.
- Pneumatic tools that shoot nails, rivets, staples, or similar fasteners, and operate at pressures more than 100 pounds per square inch (6,890 kPa), must be equipped with a special device to keep fasteners from being ejected unless the muzzle is pressed against the work surface.
- Always wear eye protection, and consider head and face protection. Set up screens whenever necessary to protect nearby workers from being struck by flying fragments around chippers, riveting guns, staplers, or air drills. A "chip guard" must be used when compressed air is used for cleaning.
- Never point compressed air guns toward anyone, and never "dead-end" them against yourself or anyone else.

Pest Control Technician Safety Manual

Liquid Fuel Tools

Fuel-powered tools are usually operated on gasoline. The most serious hazard you face when using fuel-powered tools comes from fuel vapors. They can burn, explode or poison you when you breathe them. Be careful when handling, transporting, and storing gas or other fuel. Keep away from fire, heat, and sparks. Store fuel only in containers approved for flammable liquids (see *Pesticides and Other Chemicals*).

Before refilling a fuel-powered tool tank, shut down the engine and allow it to cool to prevent accidental ignition of hazardous vapors. When you use a fuel-powered tool inside a closed area, make sure there is good ventilation or use air-supplying respirators to avoid breathing carbon monoxide. Make sure fire extinguishers are available in the area.

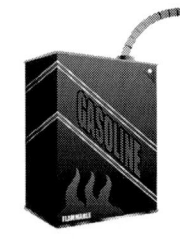

Store fuel only in approved containers

Graphic © Todd Harrison/ iStockphoto

Lasers for Bird Dispersal

A new tool in bird management is the use of lasers to disperse pest birds. The lasers are hand-held devices, looking like a radar gun or a flashlight. The operator points the laser at the birds and fires. The birds seem to view the reflected beam of light as an actual object or predator coming towards them and usually fly away.

The lasers used in bird dispersal are low-powered, but still pose some risks. A bird's eye filters out most damaging radiation, but a human's eye is unprotected from retinal tissue damage.

- Do not look into the laser.
- Lasers should not be aimed in the direction of people, roads, or aircraft.
- Particularly when using lasers in urban areas, the operator needs to consider what's behind the target area, the range of the beam, and whether the beam can reflect off of objects.

Note: Laser dispersal of birds at airports is prohibited without approval of the U.S. Federal Aviation Administration.

Jacks

All jacks, including lever and ratchet jacks, screw jacks, and hydraulic jacks, must have a stop indicator. Do not exceed the stop limit. Also, the manufacturer's load limit must be permanently marked in a prominent place on the jack. Do not exceed it.

Do not use a jack to support a lifted load for any extended period, or if you will be working underneath. In other words, once the load has been lifted, immediately block it with a jack stand or other firm and stable support.

To set up a jack, make certain of the following:

- The base of the jack rests on a firm, level surface;
- The jack is correctly centered;
- The jack head bears against a level surface; and
- The lift force is applied evenly.

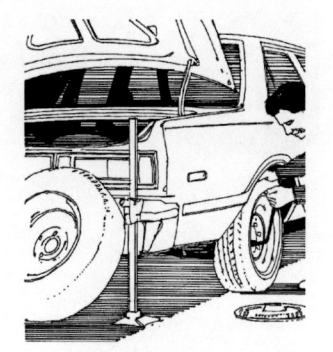

Make sure the base of the jack rests on a firm, level surface

Put a block under the base of the jack when the foundation is not firm, and place a block between the jack cap and load if the cap might slip.

Proper maintenance of jacks is essential for safety. Lubricate your jack(s) regularly, and inspect them at least once every 6 months. If a jack is subjected to abnormal loads or shock, inspect it before use and immediately thereafter.

Key Points to Remember—Hand and Power Tools

√ **Keep all tools sharp and in good condition with regular maintenance.**

√ **Examine each tool for damage before use.**

√ **Wear appropriate personal protective equipment, such as safety goggles and gloves, while using tools.**

√ **Never yank the cord or the hose to disconnect a power tool from the receptacle.**

√ **Make sure that the exposed moving parts of power tools (such as rotary saws) are safeguarded.**

√ **The third prong on the plug of a grounded tool must never be removed.**

√ **Do not use a jack to support a lifted load; once the load has been lifted, immediately block it with a jack stand or other firm support.**

√ **Do not aim bird dispersal lasers in the direction of people, roads, or aircraft.**

HEAD INJURY

The hazards you face at the job site will determine the type of protective helmet you need. While a plastic bump cap may protect you if you bang your head against a floor joist, it does not protect against penetration. A qualified hard hat, however, will even protect your head if someone on a scaffolding above drops a screwdriver. An all-purpose protective helmet must (1) absorb the shock of a blow, (2) resist penetration and in some cases, (3) protect against electrical shock.

The Occupational Safety and Health Administration (OSHA) requires that employees wear a protective helmet when working in areas where there is a potential for injury to the head from falling objects, or where there is a risk of electrical shock from exposed electrical conductors. Common sense, and often company policy, also require that you wear head protection in any situation where there is a risk of head injury. Pest control technicians wear helmets when working in crawlspaces, attics, and other tight spots, when in commercial industrial sites where employees and visitors are required to wear hard hats, and whenever there is risk from falling objects.

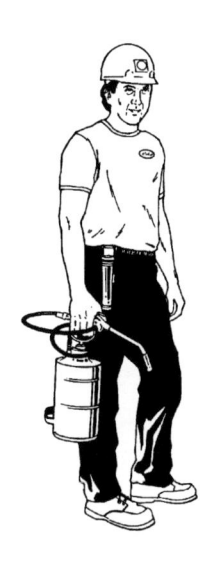

Wear a safety helmet whenever there is risk of head injury

Hard hats come in two types and three classes. Type I helmets are designed to reduce the force of a blow to the top of the head, while Type II helmets also protect against an object striking off center or to the side of the head.

The classes of hard hats are defined as follows:

♦ Class G--General. For protection against impact. Used by workers in construction, manufacturing, and lumbering, for example. Has limited voltage protection up to 2,200 volts.

♦ Class E--Electrical. For protection against electric shock up to 20,000 volts, impact, and penetration. Used by electrical and utility workers.

♦ Class C--Conductive-no electrical protection. For lightweight protection against impact. Used by construction, oil refinery, chemical plant, and other workers who are not at risk from electrical hazards.

You'll find a Class letter inside the shell of your helmet. (Note: If you have an old Class G helmet, it may be labeled Class A; an older Class E helmet may be labeled as Class B.)

Inside the helmet's molded shell is a suspension system that keeps the shell away from the wearer's skull and provides ventilation. This shock-absorbing liner consists of a headband, often with a removable sweatband, and crown straps. Plastic or vinyl straps and sweatbands are better than leather, which can absorb pesticides. Most helmets also have slots to allow you to attach hearing protectors or a face shield.

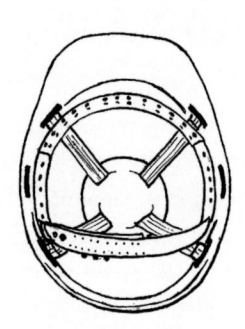

Avoid helmets with leather parts that can absorb pesticide

Key Points to Remember—Head Injury

√ *Wear a protective helmet whenever working in areas where there is a potential for injury to the head.*

√ *Wear a protective helmet where there is a risk of electrical shock from exposed electrical conductors.*

√ *Wear the proper type of helmet for the hazards faced.*

√ *Don't use a helmet with leather straps or sweatband if applying pesticides.*

HEAT AND COLD

Both heat and cold pose health hazards on the job. Our bodies are designed to work within certain temperature ranges. Raising or lowering your body temperature outside those ranges may make you sick.

Heat Illness

Perspiring is your body's way of staying cool. When you get too hot, your body puts most of its energy into cooling down. Other body functions can suffer and you'll feel the effects of heat stress. Heat illnesses range from mild heat cramps to life-threatening heat stroke.

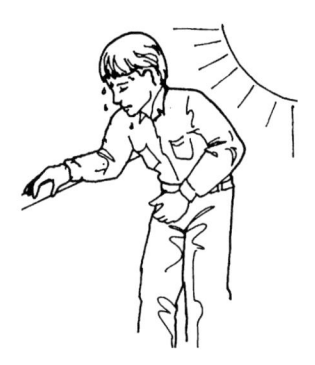

Heat illness can range from mild cramps to deadly heat stroke

You are at greater risk of heat illness if you have certain medical conditions like diabetes, or if you're overweight, or if you are taking medications like antihistamines. Working in high temperatures, high humidity and direct sunlight can be a dangerous combination. Personal protective equipment also interferes with your body's ability to perspire and cool down.

> *Precautions to Avoid Heat Illness*
> - If possible, adjust to heat by starting with short periods of work and gradually increasing the time in the heat over several days.
> - Schedule hot jobs for early or late in the day when the weather is cooler.
> - Choose personal protective equipment and clothing that is as cool as possible.
> - Outdoors, wear loose clothing, light colors, and a hat.
> - Make your own shade with a tarp or canopy. Use fans.
> - Drink plenty of water. Don't wait until you feel thirsty.
> - Schedule frequent breaks. Get into the shade.

Symptoms of Heat Illness

Mild forms of heat stress can affect your judgement on the job. You may feel weak, irritable, and less alert. You may have some or all of the following symptoms: tiredness and muscle weakness, clammy or pale skin, severe thirst, stumbling, clumsiness, dizziness, shallow breathing, headache, nausea, chills, and excessive sweating. The most serious condition, heat stroke, is characterized by mental confusion, inability to sweat, hot, dry skin, and fever. Some of these same symptoms can also indicate overexposure to certain pesticides (see *Pesticide Poisoning*).

First Aid for Heat Illness

- Stop work immediately and lie down in a cool (not cold), shady place with feet raised and clothing loosened.
- Cool down by splashing or sponging water on face, neck, and arms.
- Drink sips of cool water.

If these steps don't relieve the symptoms, or if you suspect heat stroke, notify your coworkers or your office and get medical help immediately.

Also Protect Yourself from UV Radiation in Sunlight

Skin cancer is an increasing problem. Sunlight is the main source of ultraviolet (UV) radiation known to damage skin and cause skin cancer. There are five important steps you can take to protect yourself when working outside when the UV index is high.

1. Cover up. Wear clothes to protect as much of your skin as possible.
2. Use sunscreen with an SPF of 15 or higher.
3. Wear a hat. Wide brim is best.
4. Wear sunglasses that block UV rays. Make sure they block at least 99% of both UVA and UVB radiation.
5. Limit direct sun exposure. If your shadow is shorter than you, the sun's rays are at their strongest.

Cold Weather Injuries

Cold weather injuries can range from frostnip to chilblain to hypothermia. Frostnip is a redness or swelling of surface skin. It's the first sign of impending frostbite. If frostbite occurs, the skin becomes numb, turns a waxy, grayish-white color, and is cold to the touch. Frostbite can result in permanent and serious damage to tissue.

Chilblain is an itchy inflammation caused by wet cold. Skin that is affected by chilblain is red, swollen, tender, and hot to the touch. It may itch and then become prickly or numb.

Hypothermia is a medical emergency that can be fatal. It occurs when the body's internal temperature falls below 95° F. A person suffering from hypothermia may exhibit the same symptoms as pesticide poisoning: withdrawn and bizarre behavior, irritability, confusion, slurred speech, uncoordinated movements.

Hypothermia is not just a winter problem. While it is a bigger threat when it is below freezing, hypothermia can affect you even in temperatures as high as 60° F. High wind, wet clothing, or prolonged exposure can draw the heat out of your body even in moderate weather. Certain drugs suppress the body's ability to shiver, and so make hypothermia more likely. Drugs for depression and anxiety can mask hypothermia symptoms, and alcohol can affect your judgement and so lead you to ignore those symptoms.

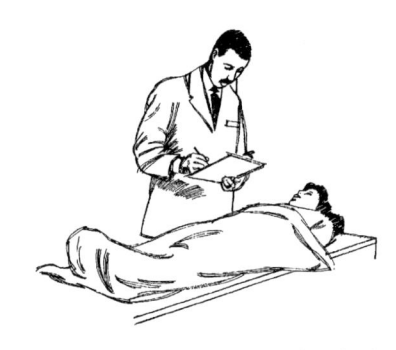

Hypothermia occurs when body temperature falls below 95° F.

All cold weather injuries, however, are more likely to occur when air temperature is below freezing (32° F). When dressing to work in cold weather, remember the acronym C.O.L.D. Keep it Clean, avoid Overheating, wear it Loose in layers, and finally, keep it Dry. It's most important to keep your head, hands, and feet dry and warm. Avoid long exposure of bare hands and wrists. Change into clean, dry socks frequently. Wear a warm hat, ideally with ear coverings. In very cold conditions, move around as much as possible to keep blood circulating.

First Aid for Cold Injuries

- Get out of the cold.
- Remove wet, constrictive clothing.
- Rewarm gradually by direct skin-to-skin contact between injured area and uninjured skin of the victim or a buddy.
- Wash and gently dry injured skin. Elevate the injured area, cover with layers of loose clothing.
- Do not pop blisters, apply lotions or creams, or massage injured area. Don't expose injured skin to extreme heat.
- Get medical attention.

Key Points to Remember—Heat and Cold

- √ You are at greater risk of heat illness if you have diabetes, are overweight, or taking medications.
- √ Heat stroke is characterized by mental confusion, inability to sweat, hot, dry skin, and fever.
- √ First aid for heat illness is: (1) Stop work immediately and lie down in a cool (not cold), shady place with feet raised and clothing loosened. (2) Cool down by splashing or sponging water on face, neck, and arms. (3) Drink sips of cool water.
- √ Cold weather injuries are more likely to occur whenever air temperature is below freezing (32° F.)
- √ A person suffering from heat stress or hypothermia may exhibit some of the same symptoms as pesticide poisoning.

HOOKWORM OR "CREEPING ERUPTION"

The name "hookworm" refers to the many species of nematodes (also called roundworms) that are intestinal parasites of animals. Two are specifically parasites of humans, but many of the animal hookworms also cause medical problems in people when they contact an infected animal's feces (typically dogs, cats, or raccoons). The results can be uncomfortable, disturbing, and even dangerous.

It is the animal hookworms that are the primary safety issue for pest control technicians working in the United States.

For most of their lives hookworms live inside the animal's intestine, sucking blood from the intestinal wall. Hookworms are typically $1/4$ to $1/3$ inch long. A mature hookworm can lay thousands of eggs a day, and there may be dozens or even hundreds of hookworms in the animal's intestine. The eggs are passed in the animal's feces, and hatch in about a week into tiny, active free-living larvae.

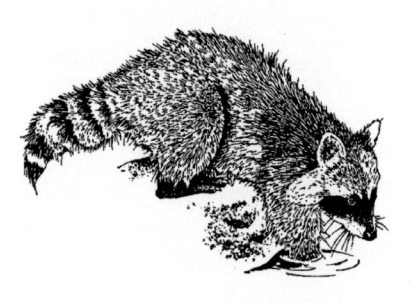

Hookworm eggs pass in animal feces and hatch into free-living larvae that may bore into the skin of people

An infective larva crawls out of the feces onto the soil surface or up onto vegetation where it stands up on its "tail" waving its head, waiting for a host. If it finds a proper host, it bores into the skin, travels through the skin to a capillary, and follows the bloodstream to the lungs. It then moves up through the trachea where it is swallowed, enters the intestinal tract, and so completes its life cycle.

A person can become infected by walking barefoot through, or eating, infected soil (the common routes of infection by children) or by crawling through infected soil with bare arms, hands, legs, etc. (the typical exposure route for technicians). The most common symptom is "creeping eruption," more properly termed "cutaneous larval migrans," inflamed, itchy tracks in the skin caused by burrowing hookworms. Because humans are an abnormal host, dog and cat hookworms are usually killed by the human immune system while still in the skin. While most human infections are mild, infection sometimes results in severe or even, very rarely, fatal disease. Raccoon roundworms are particularly nasty; they occasionally migrate to the eyes or central nervous system.

Prevention is straightforward. Do not crawl without protection (meaning coveralls, gloves, and no bare skin) in crawlspaces or other sites that may be contaminated with animal feces. Wash up thoroughly after working in such sites. If you see "creeping eruption" tracks on your skin, see a physician.

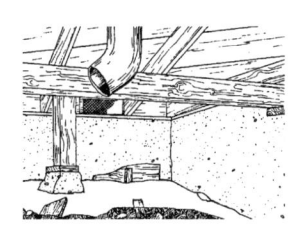

Help protect yourself from hookworm in crawlspaces by wearing coveralls and gloves

Key Points to Remember—Hookworm

- √ **People can be infected with hookworm through contact with the feces of dogs, cats, raccoons, and other animals.**
- √ **The most common symptom of hookworm is "creeping eruption," inflamed, itchy tracks in the skin caused by burrowing hookworms.**
- √ **The most common means of infection for technicians is crawling through infected soil with bare arms, hands, etc.**
- √ **Do not crawl with exposed bare skin in crawlspaces or other sites that may be contaminated with animal feces.**
- √ **Wash up thoroughly after working in such sites.**
- √ **If you see inflamed, itchy tracks on your skin, see a physician.**

HOSPITALS AND OTHER MEDICAL FACILITIES

Hospitals and other medical facilities can be hazardous places for pest control technicians. Airborne disease, medical wastes and body fluids, discarded and contaminated needles, radiation, lasers, and even violent psychiatric patients are some of the hazards which you may at times face if you work in a hospital, nursing center, or other medical facility.

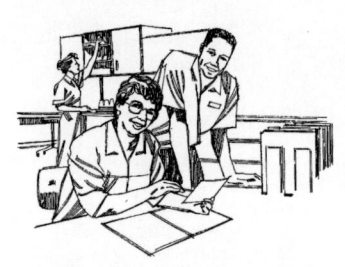

Physicians, nurses, and medical staff are trained to recognize hazards in a particular ward, treatment area, or laboratory. They know what safety precautions to follow, *and they will assume you know, as well.* Make sure you recognize and avoid the special hazards in medical areas. Do not work in areas posted as hazardous (*Biohazards, Communicable Disease, Radiation, Lasers,* etc.) without proper training, authorization, and protective equipment as necessary. Learn to recognize the different signs. If safety procedures have not been established for conducting pest control in these areas, check with those in charge to find out the specific risks on that day, and the procedures and safety precautions to follow. If you don't know what something is, do not touch it.

Hospital staff will assume that you know all about the biohazards in their area

Never reach into areas where you can't see, and never touch medical waste, blood, or body fluids (see *Bloodborne Pathogens* and *Needlesticks*). Wear the safety equipment and protective clothing that is recommended for the biohazards at each site.

And finally, do not assume someone will stop you if you are about to do something hazardous to yourself or others. At each location (ward, laboratory, etc.), check in with the person in charge to notify them of your presence and to determine whether any special precautions are necessary.

See also *Radiation* and *Tuberculosis*.

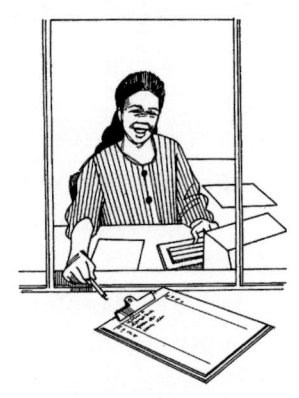

Check in first with the person in charge of each ward or laboratory

Key Points to Remember—Hospitals/Other Medical Facilities

- √ **Don't expect hospital staff to stop you from doing something stupid and dangerous.**
- √ **Check in with the person in charge at each location to notify them of your presence and to determine whether any special precautions are necessary.**
- √ **Wear the proper safety equipment and protective clothing recommended for the biohazards at each site.**
- √ **Do not work in areas posted as hazardous without express authorization and without training in the safety procedures required.**

LADDERS

Ladders pose a number of safety risks. You can fall from them, or ride them down when they fall or break. Ladders can fall off your vehicle into oncoming traffic. You can drop things from them onto other workers. You can contact live electrical lines.

Inspection

Check your ladders for obvious defects before each use. Conduct a detailed inspection of your ladders every three months or even more frequently, depending on use. For example, ladders that are carried on a truck exposed to the weather should be inspected more often. Do not use any ladders that have developed defects. Send them for repair or mark them as *"Dangerous, Do Not Use."*

Ladder Inspection

When inspecting a ladder, look for the following defects:

- splinters
- wood rot
- loose or split side rails
- loose hardware
- damaged ladder locks
- metal burrs or sharp edges
- loose or damaged rungs
- rusted metal parts
- frayed or worn ropes
- cracked or missing nonskid feet

Ladder Placement

Erect non-self-supporting ladders on a sound base with the base of the ladder a distance from the wall or upper support equal to one-quarter the length of the ladder at its point of contact. For example, if you're using a ladder that measures 20 feet from the ground to the point of support, the base of the ladder should be placed five feet (1/4 the length) away from the side of the building.

Make sure that the top of a ladder used to gain access to a roof extends at least 3 feet above the point of contact.

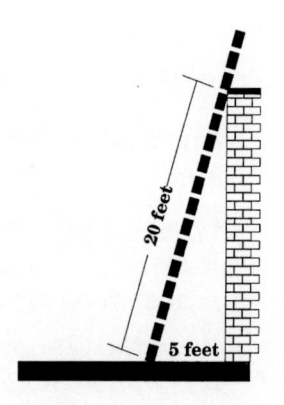

Place ladder 1/4 of its contact length away from a building and at least 3 feet above the roof

Precautions When Using Ladders

- Place the ladder on a sound base on level ground. Secure it or tie it in position.
- Use both hands on the side rails, not the rungs, to climb a ladder. Face the ladder when climbing.
- Don't carry tools or other items in your hands when going up or down a ladder. Use a tool belt, a bucket and rope, or a duffle bag to transport equipment.
- Never stand on the top three rungs of an extension ladder or the top two steps of a step ladder.
- When transporting a ladder on a vehicle, make sure it is securely attached. Then, for extra safety, add an additional safety chain or strap.
- When carrying a ladder, avoid swinging it into people or traffic.
- Wooden ladders should never be painted because paint can hide cracks or splits.
- Use only wooden or fiberglass ladders (since they are poor conductors of electricity) if you are going to be working near electrical wires or equipment.
- If you use an aluminum ladder in an area containing electrical circuits, tie off the ladder to prevent it from slipping and contacting a live electrical circuit (see *Using Ladders Around Electricity* later in this section).
- Make sure your ladders have anti-slip safety feet.

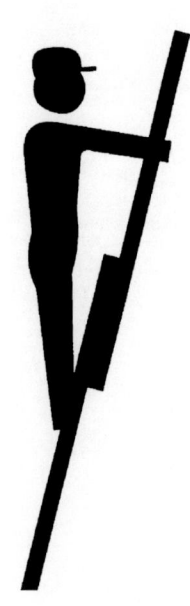

Step Ladders

Make sure that any step ladder that you use is equipped with a metal spreader or locking device of sufficient size and strength to securely hold the front and back sections in an open position. Never stand on the top two steps of a step ladder.

How to Raise and Lower an Extension Ladder

One person in good physical condition should be able to raise and lower without help an extension ladder up to 28 feet long. The key is to always keep the ladder under full control.

a) Place the ladder flat on the ground with the base against a wall.
b) Standing at the other end, raise it over your head and slowly walk towards the wall while "walking" your hands down the ladder.
c) After you have walked it all the way up against the wall, pull the base of the ladder away from the wall to conform to the recommended 4 to 1 ratio (1/4 of the ladder length from the ground to the point of support).
d) Standing directly in front of the ladder with your hand on the side rails, and blocking the base of the ladder with one foot, pull the ladder into an upright position, being careful not to pull the ladder too far over.
e) Keeping one hand on the side rail, use your stronger arm to pull the ladder rope, raising the section two or three rungs at a time before engaging the rung locks and changing your grip on the rope for the next pull.
f) Once the ladder is at the desired height, make sure the rung locks are engaged and then slowly let the ladder tip over to the wall or other support.
g) Before going up the ladder, tie the ladder rope securely around one pair of rungs on the upper and lower sections.

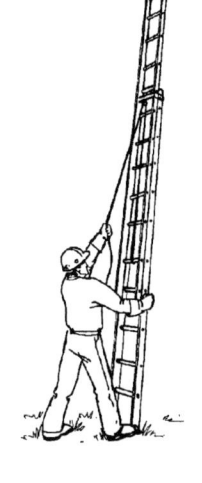

Always keep the ladder under full control

Graphic E&USA

To lower the ladder, reverse the procedure. Untie the rope, stand directly in front of the ladder, blocking the base with one foot. Pull the ladder up into an upright, balanced position, and pull on the rope to release the rung locks. Let the top section descend slowly and watch that your hand on the side rail doesn't get injured by the dropping section. Let the ladder fall gently against the wall, walk the base of the ladder back to the wall, and then walk the ladder back to the ground.

Using Ladders Around Electricity

The Consumer Product Safety Commission estimates that 65 people die each year from electrocution involving a metal ladder touching an electrical wire.

Aluminum ladders are lightweight and very popular, but they are very conductive of electricity. Wooden and fiberglass ladders are poor conductors of electricity and so are your best choices if you are going to be working around electrical wires, electrical equipment, or substations. Remember however, that *wooden and fiberglass ladders are nonconductors of electricity only when dry*. If wet, they too can conduct electricity. The Occupational Safety and Health Administration (OSHA) does allow aluminum ladders to be used in areas containing electrical circuits if proper safety measures are taken, such as securing them to prevent movement into an energized line.

Ladder electrocutions happen most often when a worker moves a ladder to a new spot without first lowering it and it touches overhead power lines. Check out the location of all overhead wires before setting up a ladder and assume that all overhead lines carry electricity. Don't try to second guess whether it's a phone line or a power line. Allow plenty of space between any overhead lines and the longest section of ladder or tool that you are using.

Before setting up or taking down ladders, a spotter should look for electrical lines and other hazards. A second technician should hold the ladder while the first technician ascends or descends. Make sure your ladder has anti-slip safety feet and tie off the ladder to keep it from slipping. Avoid using ladders on a windy day since a gust can blow the ladder into power lines.

Check out the location of all overhead wires before setting up a ladder

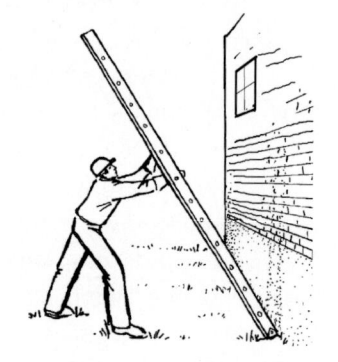

Graphic E&USA

If a ladder should start to fall into an overhead line, let it go. Never try to move it off of the line. Have someone call the power company while you stand guard to make sure that no one touches the ladder. Be sure the power company cuts off the power before the ladder is moved.

If someone is touching a ladder when it comes in contact with electricity, don't try to pull them away with your hands. Use something that does not conduct electricity like a dry piece of wood to push or pull the person loose.

Ladder electrocutions can also occur when a technician touches an electrical source such as an exterior light socket or if he is handling an improperly grounded power tool while on a ladder.

There's yet another type of ladder electrical hazard--lightning. If there's lightning in the area, get off of that roof or out of that tree, pronto (see *Electric Shock*).

Key Points to Remember—Ladders

- √ **Use wooden or fiberglass ladders if you are going to be working around electrical wires or equipment.**
- √ **Erect non-self-supporting ladders with the base of the ladder a distance from the wall or upper support equal to one-quarter the length of the ladder.**
- √ **Make sure that the top of a ladder used to gain access to a roof extends at least 3 feet above the point of contact.**
- √ **Inspect your ladders frequently.**
- √ **Never stand on the top three rungs of an extension ladder or the top two steps of a step ladder.**
- √ **When transporting a ladder in a vehicle, make sure it is securely attached.**
- √ **Know the proper procedure to raise and lower an extension ladder by yourself.**
- √ **Check out the location of overhead wires before setting up or moving a ladder.**

LIFTING AND BACK SAFETY

Protect your back. Back injuries account for almost 1/3 of service-related illnesses and injuries that cause days off work. Back injuries are among the most expensive for businesses and the most painful for workers. Back injuries generally involve more time convalescing and require more therapy than other injuries. Chronic back injuries are the major cause of workers' compensation claims.

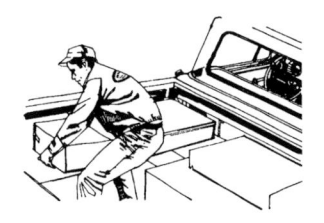

Lift properly, watch your posture, and do regular back strengthening exercises

The best way you can prevent injury to your back is to lift properly, watch your posture and do regular back-strengthening exercises.

The number one rule for proper lifting is to *"Think Before You Lift."* Slow down and lift the load mentally first. If you're not sure you can lift the load by yourself, don't be a hero. Get help from another person or, if you can't find another person, use a dolly or hand truck.

- Face the object you're going to lift. Plant your feet evenly, close to the object.
- Don't bend from the waist with your legs locked. Bend your knees and take advantage of your more powerful thigh muscles to help lift the load.
- Lift and move slowly and evenly. Avoid jerky movements or twisting your body.
- Hold a heavy load close to your body, not out at arm's length.
- Don't lift a heavy load higher than your waist.
- If two people are lifting a heavy load, only one should direct the movements.
- Before you lift, make sure you have a place to set the load down.
- Reverse the lifting process to set the load down. Keeping your back straight, slowly bend your knees and set the load down gradually.

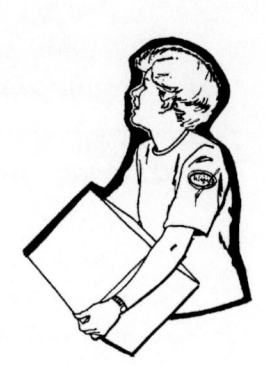

Hold a heavy load close to your body

Key Points to Remember—Lifting and Back Safety

√ **The number one rule regarding lifting is to "Think Before You Lift."**

√ **If you're not sure you can lift the load by yourself, get help from another person, or use a dolly or hand truck.**

√ **Don't lift a heavy load higher than your waist.**

√ **Before you lift, make sure you have a place to set the load down.**

LOCKOUT/TAGOUT

Before a worker services or maintains a machine or piece of equipment that uses or releases "hazardous energy," OSHA requires that it first be isolated from its energy source, and then locked or tagged. Hazardous energy refers to electrical, mechanical, hydraulic, pneumatic, chemical, and heat energy as well as air, gas, or steam pressure. Isolating the equipment from its energy source can mean disconnecting circuits, releasing pressure, closing valves, even blocking elevated machine parts to keep them from moving.

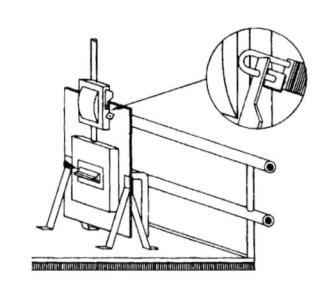

Lockout is using a lock or a bolt to physically prevent anyone from turning on a machine

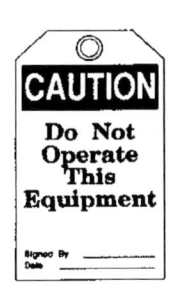

Lockout refers to actually locking or bolting the disconnect switch or valve after the machine has been shut down so that no one can mistakenly turn it on. For example, a worker would switch off a circuit breaker for a conveyor belt and then put a padlock on the breaker box before working under the conveyor. Lockout is a more secure way of making sure that no one is injured and should be used whenever possible. If there is no way to lock the switch, circuit box, or valves, then tagout must be used instead.

Tags warn of danger but do not prevent operation of equipment

Tagout means placing a special warning tag or sign on the disconnect switch or valve that reads something like, "DANGER —Do Not Open Valve," or "DANGER—Do Not Start This Motor." Tags warn employees of danger but don't actually prevent operation of the equipment. Additional safety measures must be used if equipment is tagged instead of locked.

How does this affect pest control technicians? Contractors are covered under this OSHA Standard. So a pest control technician treating or working around a piece of equipment that could start up or release energy and cause injury is subject to the lockout/tagout rules of the business he or she is servicing.

Do not remove lockout devices or tags, and never restart equipment that is locked out or tagged. Only specially trained, authorized employees can do so. If a lockout device

Never restart equipment that has been locked or tagged

needs to be removed or a tagged piece of equipment operated, find the authorized employee that can do so. The locks and tags must identify the authorized employee who placed them.

Lockout/tagout operations are the responsibility of the commercial customer. But technicians must understand them. Any company that is required to use lockout/tagout procedures must notify its contractors of those procedures.

Key Points to Remember—Lockout/Tagout

- √ *Lockout refers to actually locking or bolting the disconnect switch or valve after the machine has been shut down so that no one can mistakenly turn it on.*
- √ *Tagout means placing a special warning tag or sign on the disconnect switch or valve.*
- √ *If you work around a piece of equipment that could start up or release energy and cause injury you are subject to any lockout/tagout rules.*
- √ *In a facility with lockout/tagout rules in place, equipment cannot be operated until locks or tags are removed by an authorized employee.*

MOLDS

Molds are the most common forms of fungi found on the earth. Most reproduce through the formation of spores, tiny microscopic cells that float through the indoor and outdoor air on a continual basis. We are all exposed to mold spores in the air we breathe on a daily basis.

Molds are found almost everywhere in our environment, both outdoors and indoors. They can grow on just about any substance, as long as moisture and oxygen are available. Mold growth may occur when excessive moisture accumulates in buildings or on building materials including carpet, ceiling tile, insulation, paper, wallboard, wood, surfaces behind wallpaper, or in heat-

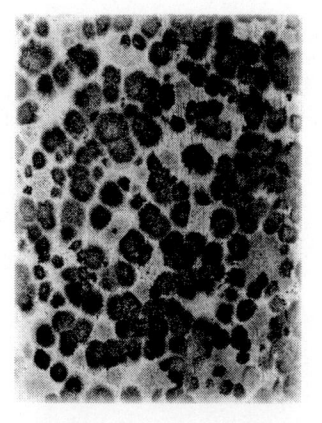

Mold colonies growing on a wall inside a home

Photo © Shaun Lowe/iStockphoto

ing, ventilation, and air conditioning (HVAC) systems, and in crawlspaces and attics. It can also grow on grains and other stored bulk foods in commercial food and agriculture operations. An earthy or musty odor is an indication of mold growth.

Health Effects

Molds can cause three types of adverse health effects in humans: allergy, infection, and toxin-mediated conditions. The critical factors which determine a mold's health impact are the extent of the mold infestation, the airborne concentration of contaminants, and the sensitivity of the individuals exposed.

Most people experience no health effects from exposure to the molds present in indoor or outdoor air. However, some individuals with underlying health conditions may be more sensitive to molds. For example, individuals who have other allergies or existing respiratory conditions such as asthma, sinusitis, or other lung diseases may be more easily affected. Similarly, persons who have a weakened immune system tend to be more sensitive to molds.

> *Common Health Effects from Mold Exposure*
>
> The most common health effects associated with mold exposure include allergic reactions similar to common pollen or animal allergies. Symptoms include sneezing, runny nose, eye irritation, coughing, congestion, aggravation of asthma, and skin rash.

In rare instances, serious conditions can arise after mold exposure. These effects occur most often in people who are health-compromised in some way, but also to otherwise healthy individuals who are exposed to very high levels of mold or mold spores. Examples include pneumonitis, other infections, and various toxic reactions to the chemical by-products produced in molds. These by-products are called "mycotoxins."

Toxic Mold

The phrase "toxic mold" has been used by journalists and many others to refer to molds that have been implicated in severe health effects in humans. Although not a scientific term, it is typically used in the press to refer to those molds capable of producing mycotoxins and incorrectly implies that these molds are more dangerous than others. In fact, all molds under the right conditions have the potential to cause allergic reactions, infections, and toxic reactions.

Stachybotrys chartarum (also known as *Stachybotrys atra*) is the mold associated with most lawsuits. *Stachybotrys* is a greenish-black mold that grows on materials with high cellulose and low nitrogen content. Like other molds, it requires a water source from high humidity, water leaks, heavy condensation, or flooding. It's known for growing behind walls and beneath floors. Typical mold growth sites are fiberboard, gypsum board, paper, ceiling tiles, wallpaper, cotton fabric, carpet backing, dust, lint, and wooden construction elements.

Potential Mold Exposure for Pest Control Technicians

All of us are exposed to mold at home and at work. Mold grows on the grout in our showers and on our basement walls; mold spores float in the air of our homes. Crawlspaces and basements are the areas most likely to have moisture levels high enough to support mold. But you can be exposed to mold or mold spores whenever you work in an area that has a moisture problem, or that has had one in the past.

Technicians doing moisture control work have the highest potential exposure to molds, particularly when removing water-damaged materials.

Technicians working in grain storage facilities also have a higher exposure risk from molds growing on damp or spoiled grain or forage.

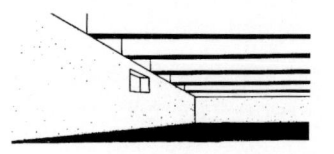

Mold often grows in wet crawlspaces and basements

(*Farmer's lung disease* is the name given to hypersensitivity pneumonitis caused by an allergic reaction to molds found in spoiled grain or forage products.)

Personal Protection Against Mold

Since there are no existing standards regarding personal protective equipment for mold inspection, follow the guidelines established for working around asbestos.

As with asbestos protection, match your protective equipment with the degree of potential exposure. If you are doing work with a higher risk of mold exposure, such as mold inspections or removing water-damaged materials where mold is present, or if you simply believe there is a high risk of mold, be sure to wear goggles, coveralls, and an OSHA-approved N-95 or better particulate respirator (not a cheap dust mask). In some instances you may want to wear a respirator with a 100-level high efficiency (HE) rating.

When working in a crawlspace or other area with a high mold potential, protect your customers as well as yourself. Disturbance will increase the number of mold spores in the air, so turn off the air handler or create a negative pressure with fans, so that any spores driven up into the air will not be circulated into living areas.

If you are removing water-damaged materials that have since dried out, wet them down first with water or a disinfectant solution to minimize airborne mold contamination.

Key Points to Remember—Mold

- √ **All molds under the right conditions have the potential to cause allergic reactions, infections, and toxic reactions.**
- √ **The health risk from exposure to mold is determined by the extent of the mold infestation, the airborne concentration of contaminants, and the sensitivity of the individuals exposed.**
- √ **You can be exposed to mold or mold spores whenever you work in an area that has a moisture problem, or that has had one in the past.**
- √ **When there is a high risk of mold, be sure to wear goggles, coveralls, and an OSHA-approved N-95 or better particulate respirator.**

NATURAL GAS

Natural gas is a combustible mixture of hydrocarbon gases. While natural gas is formed primarily of methane (70%-90%), it can also include ethane, propane, butane and pentane. It is colorless and odorless in its pure form. Of course, its most important characteristic is that it is combustible, and when burned it gives off a great deal of energy.

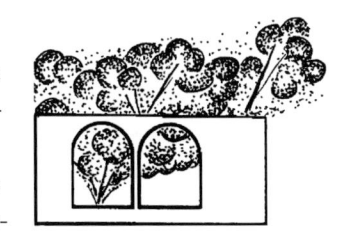

Natural gas is explosive when it builds up in an enclosed space

Natural gas can also be massively explosive when it builds up in an enclosed space and ignites. Everyone has seen the result of those rare natural gas explosions on the evening news.

Since it has no odor of its own, an odorant is added as a warning. The "rotten-egg" smell is mercaptan or a similar sulfur-based compound that can be easily detected by most people at a level well below the flammability level of natural gas.

ALERT: People who have a diminished sense of smell may not be able to smell the warning agent added to natural gas.

Gas leaks can occur inside in or near appliances, or outdoors from buried gas pipes.

Common signs of a gas leak include:

- A gas odor (which can best be described as the smell of rotten eggs)
- A blowing or hissing sound
- Water bubbling or being blown into the air at a pond, creek, or river
- Dirt being blown or thrown into the air
- Fire coming from the ground or burning above the ground
- Unusual brown or dead patches of vegetation on or near a pipeline location
- A dry spot in a moist field

If You Smell Natural Gas...

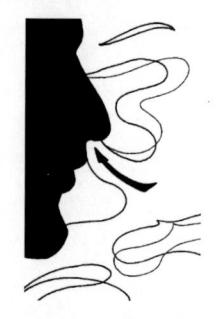

If the gas odor is very weak, most likely a pilot light is out and needs to be relit. Do not relight it yourself. Notify the tenant, owner, or manager. If the gas odor is strong, or if you hear a hissing or blowing sound, don't attempt to locate the problem. *Do not do anything that could create a spark.* Alert others and leave the building immediately. On the way out:

- Do **NOT** light a match or a cigarette lighter.
- Do **NOT** turn any appliance on or off.
- Do **NOT** use the phone.
- Do **NOT** turn any electrical switches on or off.
- Do **NOT** use a flashlight.
- **DO** leave the door open.
- **DO** warn others to stay away.

If you smell rotting eggs, it may signal a natural gas leak

If the property owner is not present, as soon as you are safely away from the building, call your office. Have them notify the fire department and gas company. If you cannot reach your office or the property owner, call the fire department and gas company yourself. Remember, do not reenter the building to use the phone.

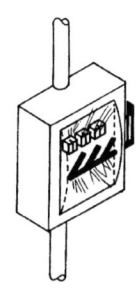

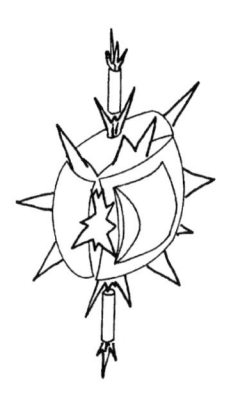

Arcs and sparks occur inside switches and equipment; if you smell natural gas, do not turn anything on or off

Gas Connectors on Appliances

The biggest hazard to pest control technicians from natural gas comes from pest control work in, around, and under gas appliances, most often stoves but also furnaces, heat pumps, space heaters, water heaters, fireplaces, outdoor gas lights, and dryers.

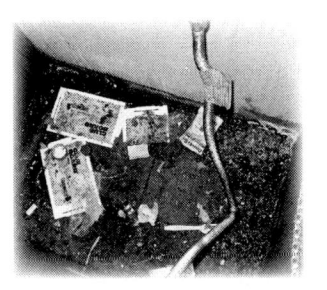

Connectors on gas stoves that are frequently pulled out for cleaning or service are under great stress

Be careful if you pull out gas stoves or gas dryers for inspection or treatment. Old, corroded, or too-short corrugated gas connectors can break. The older the connector, the greater the possibility of failure, and in pest control we often work around very old appliances.

According to the Consumer Product Safety Commission, some of the uncoated brass connectors which were used many years ago have a flaw that can cause a leak, fire, or explosion. These brass connectors haven't been made for 25 years, but they may still be in use in older homes and apartments. Because of these risks, many companies do not permit technicians to move gas appliances. Check with your supervisor.

> **ALERT:** In apartments, it's best to have maintenance staff or an authorized individual pull appliances for you. Some state and local regulations require a gasfitter's or plumber's license to move any natural gas appliance.

If you're working around a gas appliance and smell a strong smell of gas or hear a hissing or blowing sound:

1. Follow the rules listed above under "If You Smell Natural Gas..."
2. Close the appliance shut-off valve, if nearby, but only if you can do so without moving the appliance or disturbing the connector.
3. Evacuate everyone from the building immediately, opening doors and windows as you go, and leaving the front door open when you leave.

Key Points to Remember—Natural Gas

- √ **If you smell a strong gas odor, or hear a hissing sound, alert others and leave the building immediately.**
- √ **Do not do anything that could create a spark.**
- √ **Do not turn any electrical switches on or off, even on a flashlight.**
- √ **Use a telephone _away_ from the building to call for emergency help from the fire department or gas company.**

NEEDLESTICKS

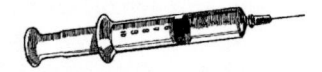

There are about 800,000 accidental "needlesticks" each year. About 2 percent of used needles are contaminated with HIV that can cause AIDS, even more with hepatitis B and C. These diseases and others can be transmitted by accidental needlesticks. Nurses, physicians, and other medical professionals experience roughly two thirds of needlestick injuries, but others are at risk. Housekeepers, maintenance workers, and service personnel, such as pest control technicians, are at risk when working in medical facilities, as well as around sites of illegal drug use.

Imagine this: while inspecting a sick person's room, you reach under the bed. Ouch! Something sticks you in the finger. It's a used needle (syringe) that someone has dropped. Then you learn the sick person is suffering from AIDS. Is that a frightening thought?

The risk that a pest control technician will become infected with hepatitis or HIV from a needlestick is admittedly low. But maintenance workers and other non-medical people have been infected just that way.

Minimize your risk. Be alert to discarded needles under beds and furniture, inside cabinets and drawers, and in trash cans, particularly when working in medical facilities, in rooms with sick people, or in high-crime/drug use locations. *Never reach into areas where you can't see, such as under the bed.* If you work in patient areas of medical facilities, be sure to understand and follow any safety procedures recommended. Such procedures might include wearing Kevlar® gloves (see box) or two pairs of medical gloves, a practice called "double-gloving" (see *Bloodborne Pathogens*).

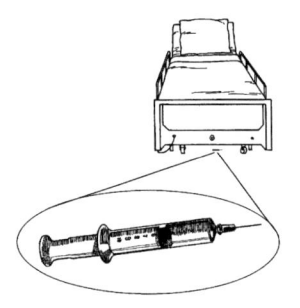

Never reach into areas where you can not see, such as under a bed

Kevlar® Gloves May Help Prevent Needlesticks

Some military installations are requiring that their pest control technicians wear Kevlar® gloves to help protect from needlesticks (among other things). Police wear Kevlar gloves for the same reasons. Kevlar is the material used in body armor and is quite cut, tear, and puncture-resistant. One experimental lab study estimated that Kevlar gloves were 15 times as effective as latex gloves at preventing needlestick transmission of HIV.

Pest control technicians at military installations often use police leather gloves lined with Kevlar, which run around $35 a pair at police supply stores. Intermediate Kevlar gloves (such as those used in the lab study) are less expensive at $7-10 per pair.

Pest control technicians are increasingly finding discarded syringes in crawlspaces and basements during inspections. Homeless people and drug addicts may use these sites if they are accessible from the outside of a building or if they are not locked from the inside.

When crawling such locations, heavy duty leather gloves or medical gloves are a good idea, as well as rubber knee pads. Make sure you have a good flashlight when moving through a crawlspace or basement and shine the light on each area before you enter it. Move slowly, take your time, and don't reach into any dark corners without lighting them first.

First Aid After a Needlestick

(1) <u>Immediately</u> wash and disinfect the wound.
(2) Inform the appropriate medical supervisor (if in a medical facility) or facility manager and call your office.
(3) Save the needle so it can be tested.
(4) Notify your physician.

Note: Steps 1-4 should be done as quickly as possible. Do not delay.

(5) Write down the details of how the exposure occurred.
(6) Get yourself tested for hepatitis and HIV.
(7) Make sure that someone at your company makes arrangements to have the source individual (the person whose needle it was) tested to determine whether they are HIV or hepatitis positive.

Key Points to Remember—Needlesticks

√ **Used needles can transmit HIV (which causes AIDS), hepatitis, and other diseases.**

√ **Be alert to discarded needles under beds and furniture, inside cabinets and drawers, and in trash cans.**

√ **Never reach into areas where you can't see, such as under a bed.**

√ **If you are stuck by a used needle, <u>immediately</u> wash and disinfect the wound, notify the proper supervisor, save the needle, and get medical advice.**

NOISE

Pest control technicians face some risk of hearing damage in certain situations, such as using hammer drills in termite control, operating certain types of fogging equipment, and working in food plants and other industrial sites.

> *Key Facts About Noise*
> - Exposure to loud sounds can cause hearing loss.
> - Noise intensity is measured in decibels (dB). A decibel is a unit that measures the intensity of sound on a scale from zero to 140. Normal breathing measures about 10dB, conversation about 60dB, and shouting directly in someone's ear, 110dB.
> - The scale is logarithmic--90dB is 10 times louder than 80dB.
> - In general, the higher the decibels (the louder the noise), the quicker the injury.
> - Noise duration is also critical. To know if a sound is loud enough to damage your ears, it is important to know both the loudness level and the length of exposure to the sound.
> - Sounds louder than 85dB can damage your ears, depending on the length of exposure.
> - Drilling concrete with a hammer drill typically produces a noise level between 90 and 95dB. Four to eight hours of this, without some sort of hearing protection, can cause injury.
> - The average chain saw at full throttle produces a noise level of about 105dB. This noise level is high enough to cause eventual hearing loss if sustained for more than one hour without hearing protection.

Reducing the Volume or Duration of the Noise

The longer you are exposed to a loud noise, the more damaging it may be. The louder the noise, the higher the risk. Also, the closer you are to the source of intense noise, the more damaging it is. (Every gunshot produces a noise that could damage the ears of anyone in close hearing range.)

So, to protect your ears, you either reduce the length of your exposure to a loud noise, or you reduce the noise level. You can reduce the noise level either by increasing your distance from the source of the noise, or by wearing special hearing protection.

Pest Control Technician Safety Manual

There are two common styles of hearing protectors: ear muffs and ear plugs. One or the other may be more suitable in certain work environments.

Ear Muffs

Ear muffs cover the ears and fit over the top of the head. They tend to offer better sound protection but they may be uncomfortable in a hot, humid environment. If you must wear a bump cap or hard hat on the job, there are ear muff attachments that clip onto the cap. There are also special ear muffs for people who wear glasses. Ear muffs may be a better choice for people with unusually shaped ear canals who may find ear plugs uncomfortable.

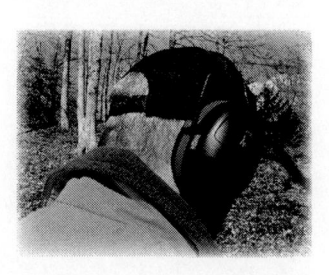

Ear muffs typically offer better sound protection

Ear Plugs

Ear plugs are inserted into the ear canal. (Note: Cotton balls are not considered an acceptable protective device.) Ear plugs come as either one-size-fits-all, molded in several sizes, or as formable plugs that expand to fit the ear canal. Reusable ear plugs need to be cleaned and disinfected regularly to reduce risk of infection. Ear plugs may be connected with a cord to prevent their loss and so that they can be worn around your neck when not in use.

Noise Reduction Rating (NRR)

A hearing protection device reduces the noise to an acceptable level, it does not block all sound, so if the noise is loud enough, regular hearing protection may not be adequate to prevent injury. The Noise Reduction Rating (NRR) is the measure, in decibels, of how well a hearing protector reduces noise. The NRR will be listed on the package or on the device itself.

The higher the number, the greater the noise reduction. Ear plugs with an NRR of 30 reduce a dangerous 100dB noise down to a safe 70dB (100dB - 30dB = 70dB).

The best noise reduction rating of a hearing protector is one high enough to reduce noise to an acceptable level, but still low enough for you to hear vocal commands while on the job.

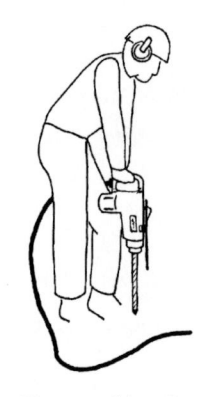

Use good hearing protection when using a hammer drill or other loud equipment

| 106 |

Key Points to Remember—Noise

√ **Loud noises can cause hearing loss.**

√ **Wear hearing protection devices such as ear muffs or ear plugs whenever noise exceeds safe levels.**

√ **If the noise is loud enough, hearing protection may not be adequate to prevent injury.**

√ **Reusable ear plugs need to be cleaned and disinfected regularly to reduce risk of infection.**

PESTICIDES AND OTHER CHEMICALS

Many of the chemicals you work with on a day-to-day basis are poisons, they are toxic to you in some way or another. Pesticides are the best example. While they are designed to kill pests...insects, rodents, or whatever...they are toxic to people, as well. Who is most at risk from the pesticides you use? You are, because you handle those pesticides every day. You also face risks from other chemicals at work; examples include gasoline and solvents.

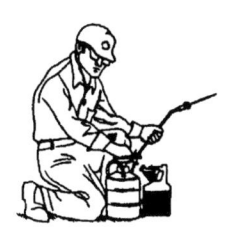

You are the one most at risk from pesticide exposure

Hazard Communication Standard

The Occupational Safety and Health Administration, commonly called OSHA, is part of the U.S. Department of Labor. OSHA sets *standards* to protect workers on-the-job. The *Hazard Communication Standard* is designed to give you the information you need to protect yourself from hazardous chemicals, including the pesticides you use at work. Its purpose is to reduce the incidence of chemically-caused illnesses and injuries in the workplace.

The *Hazard Communication Standard* is based on these simple concepts:

(1) You, as an employee, have a need and a right to know the hazards and identities of the chemicals, such as pesticides, you might be exposed to when working.

(2) You also need to know what protective measures are available to prevent any illness and injury from these hazardous chemicals.

Pest Control Technician Safety Manual

Legal Requirements of the Hazard Communication Standard

OSHA requires that you be informed about the following legal requirements of OSHA's *Hazard Communication Standard*:

- A company must have a written list of all hazardous chemicals in the workplace. This list will include not only all pesticides but solvents, gasoline, and cleaning fluids.
- A company must obtain a material safety data sheet (MSDS) for each hazardous chemical (see below). You and other employees must have ready access to the MSDSs.
- Containers of hazardous materials must be labeled, tagged, or marked with the identity of the chemical and appropriate hazard warnings. Manufacturer's labels are preferred. If a chemical is transferred to another container, the new container must be labeled.
- All workers who may be exposed to hazardous materials must be provided information and training prior to working with or around those materials. Among other things, you should be trained about the hazards of the chemicals you use, how to protect yourself from those hazards, how to use personal protective equipment (PPE) how to read labels and MSDSs, and how to obtain and use hazard information.
- A company must have a formal Hazard Communication Program, and it must be in writing. The program identifies responsible individuals, includes the list of hazardous chemicals (see above), and discusses procedures and methods for compliance with the *Hazard Communication Standard*.

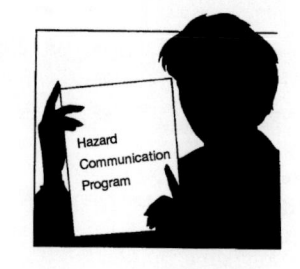

A company hazard communication program describes how employees will be protected from chemicals

MSDS

A **M**aterial **S**afety **D**ata **S**heet, called an MSDS for short, is a quick guide to the potential hazards of a pesticide or other chemical. Although an MSDS has some of the same information that you can find on a pesticide label, it also provides details about the pesticide's chemistry, toxicology, and health and environmental hazards, as well as instructions on what to do after a spill or other emergency. An MSDS usually refers to the concentrated material, just as it comes from the package. It is primarily designed for workers who use or may be exposed to the chemical. The Occupational Safety and Health Administration (OSHA) requires that the manufacturer or distributor of each hazardous chemical develop and distribute an MSDS for that product. Employers are required to make MSDSs available to every employee selling, storing, or handling the product. By law, each Material Safety Data Sheet must include certain information, although the section headings and their order may vary:

Identification and Ingredients

- **Product Identification.** Identifies the chemical along with any trade names or common names. Also gives manufacturer's name and address, and may include an emergency phone number.
- **Hazardous Ingredients.** Lists the individual hazardous ingredients in the product. Shows the maximum concentration of each ingredient to which someone may be safely exposed.

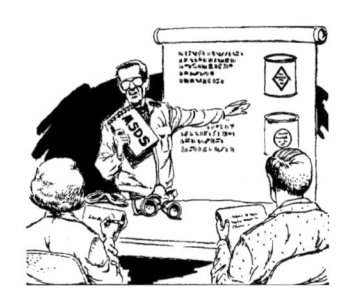

An MSDS provides details about a chemical, including health and environmental hazards

- **Physical Characteristics.** Describes the chemical product's color, odor, and general appearance. Also contains technical information on the product's boiling point, solubility in water, vapor pressure, and the like.

Potential Hazards

- **Fire and Explosion Information.** Tells you at what temperature the product will ignite (see discussion of pesticide flash point in *Fire*), and what materials to use to extinguish a fire. Describes any unusual fire or explosion hazards and special fire fighting procedures and equipment that may be necessary.
- **Reactivity Information.** Tells whether the chemical will react dangerously when mixed with something else or exposed to certain conditions. The "incompatibility" section identifies other chemicals that, when combined, can cause a dangerous reaction. The "instability" section describes the environmental conditions (such as heat or bright light) that could cause a dangerous reaction.
- **Health Information.** Includes a list of symptoms of overexposure such as headache, dizziness, skin rash, nausea. Lists any medical conditions that

might be aggravated by overexposure to the chemical. Provides first aid and emergency information in case of poisoning.

Safety Recommendations

- **Spill, Leak, and Storage Procedures.** Tells you how to clean up a spill or leak, special precautions to take, and what materials to use for cleanup. Describes ways to dispose of the spilled product. Proper storage procedures may be detailed in this section or in the *Special Precautions* section.
- **Personal Protection.** Lists the protective equipment (such as rubber gloves, goggles, respirator) needed in order to safely handle the chemical. May also include information on aerating a treatment site or ventilating a storage area.
- **Special Precautions.** A catchall section for information not covered elsewhere. May include additional safety and health precautions when handling the material. This section may also list hazards to birds, fish, wildlife, and the environment.

Toxicity

Toxicity is the degree to which a chemical is poisonous. It is a physical characteristic of a material just like its boiling point. The more toxic a chemical is, the less of it is required to do damage.

LD_{50}

Before a pesticide can be registered, the manufacturer has to determine its toxicity; specifically, just how much of the pesticide it takes to cause illness or death to people, pets, and other nontarget animals. Tests are run on laboratory animals, particularly rats and mice.

LD_{50} is scientific shorthand for Lethal Dose to 50% of the test animals. The test chemical is eaten by the animals (acute oral LD_{50}) or absorbed through the skin (acute dermal LD_{50}). The number is given in mg/kg--the number of milligrams of toxicant per kilogram of body weight. So, if you gave a dose of a chemical equal to its LD_{50} to a group of 10 laboratory rats, you would expect 5 of those rats to die.

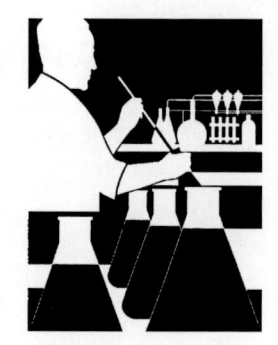

The lower the LD50, the more toxic the pesticide

A pesticide's LD_{50} number is more useful to a chemist than to a pest control technician. Nevertheless, LD_{50}s often appear on MSDSs, in training literature, and on certification exams. The important things to remember about LD_{50}s are these:

- The most practical use for LD_{50} is simply to compare relative toxicity between products. But be sure you are not comparing apples and oranges. An LD_{50} value can be for the formulation concentrate or for the end-use dilution. It can be for absorption (dermal), or consumption (oral). These numbers will be quite different.
- The lower the LD_{50} number, the more poisonous is the pesticide. For example, a chemical with an LD_{50} of 80 mg/kg is much more toxic than one with an LD_{50} that is greater than 5,000 mg/kg.
- The LD_{50} determines, to a large extent, the *signal word* and *precautionary statements* on a pesticide's label. The least acutely toxic products get a "caution" label, those of intermediate toxicity get a "warning" label, and those that are highly toxic get a "danger" label (see below).
- The LD_{50} value provides information only about acute, short-term toxic effects, not long-term exposure.

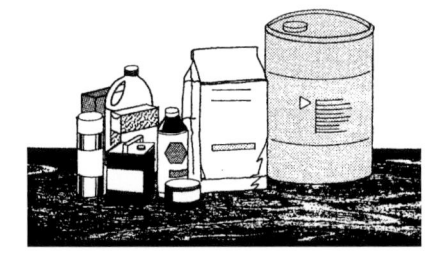

All pesticides pose some degree of risk. None are completely safe

Signal Words

Pesticides are grouped into categories based on how toxic they are to people, animals, and the environment. Special identifying words--called "signal words"--are printed in large letters on every pesticide label to show how toxic the product is. The signal words are DANGER, WARNING, and CAUTION.

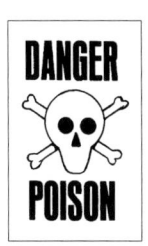

Pesticide products labeled DANGER are highly toxic. If the concentrate was swallowed, as little as a taste to a teaspoonful could kill the average person. All highly toxic pesticides that are very likely to cause acute illness through oral, dermal, or inhalation exposure, also will carry the word POISON printed in red and the skull and crossbones symbol. Products that have the signal word DANGER due to skin and eye irritation potential will not carry the word POISON or the skull and crossbones symbol.

WARNING

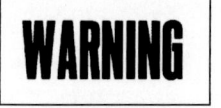

Pesticide products labeled WARNING are moderately toxic. They may cause acute illness from oral, dermal, or inhalation exposure, or they are likely to cause moderate skin or eye irritation. The fatal oral dose for the concentrate is estimated to be between one and three teaspoonfuls.

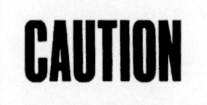

CAUTION

Pesticide products labeled CAUTION are slightly toxic or relatively nontoxic and have only slight potential to cause illness or skin or eye irritation.

No matter what the signal word, however, there is no pesticide that is absolutely safe. All pose some degree of risk.

Applicator Risks by Formulation

Pesticide formulations used by pest control technicians pose little risk when handled properly. Even so, certain formulations present more of a hazard to the applicator than others. The list below is a general guideline. Individual products may have more or less, or a different hazard to the applicator than indicated here. Check the "Precautionary Statements" section of the pesticide label before mixing and using the product.

Aerosols

- Inhalation hazard during application, especially in confined spaces
- Hazard to eyes from splashback
- Propellants in some pressurized aerosol containers are flammable and must be kept from heat, flame, or puncture

Baits

- Little hazard to applicator

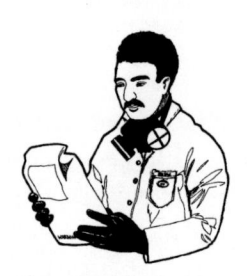

Dusts

- Inhalation hazard filling equipment and during application
- May irritate eyes, nose, throat, and skin
- Potential eye hazard from abrasive particles

Check the "Precautionary Statements" before mixing or using a pesticide

Emulsifiable Concentrates
- Some undiluted products are flammable
- Skin absorption is faster, as a rule, than with wettable powders or other dry formulations
- Hazard to eyes from splashback
- Finished mix conducts electricity

Granules
- Little hazard to applicator

Microencapsulates
- Finished mix conducts electricity
- Hazard to eyes from splashback

Wettable Powder
- Inhalation hazard during mixing (although water-soluble packets eliminate this risk)
- Usually little risk of skin absorption (however, the packaging of some wettable powders makes them hard to mix without getting on the skin, and so absorption through hands becomes a risk)
- Finished mix conducts electricity

Gasoline

You use gasoline in your vehicle and probably in gasoline-powered equipment, as well. Gasoline is a hazardous material. First, and foremost, it is extremely flammable. Gasoline ignites easily and burns vigorously. Gasoline vapor may explode. Second, exposure to gasoline liquid or vapor can make you sick. The material safety data sheet (MSDS) for gasoline provides this overview of the product's hazards:

- Extremely flammable
- Harmful or fatal if swallowed-- can enter lungs and cause damage
- Vapor harmful
- May cause eye and skin irritation
- Long-term exposure to vapor has caused cancer in laboratory animals
- Keep out of reach of children

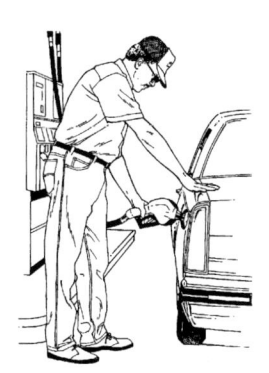

Gasoline may be the most dangerous chemical you use

Pest Control Technician Safety Manual

Precautions With Gasoline

Unless you are a fumigator, gasoline is the most dangerous material you use. Unfortunately, most of us are so familiar with gasoline that we tend to ignore its hazards. Don't be careless; follow these safety precautions:

- Avoid breathing gasoline fumes.
- Make sure gasoline is not near any heat source or flame.
- Store only in approved containers.
- Inspect portable gas containers before use. The inside should be free of dirt and debris and the cap should form a tight seal capable of preventing the escape of either vapor or liquid. Metal containers should be free of corrosion. Plastic containers should be free of stress cracks.
- Avoid storing a gasoline container in a vehicle. Do not place gasoline in the passenger compartment.
- When filling portable containers, remove the container from the vehicle, place it on the ground a safe distance from the vehicle, and follow proper safety procedures (see *Precautions When Filling Gas Cans* in *Driving and Vehicle Safety*).

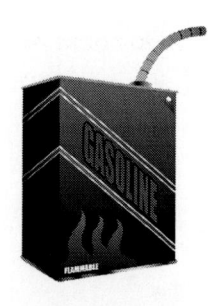

Gasoline ignites easily, burns vigorously, and may explode

> **WARNING**—Gasoline vapor is invisible and heavier than air. It can flow along the pavement for some distance when not dispersed by air currents. If ignited, the vapor becomes a fuse that brings the flame back to the liquid gasoline source. The distance that is "safe" depends on the conditions, but fire experts believe placing the container about five feet from an ignition source usually should be sufficient.

- Put out cigarettes or cigars before fueling.
- Before putting a container of gasoline in the trunk of a vehicle, or in the bed of a pickup or truck, tighten the cap of the container and the cap of the air vent, if there is one. Wipe the outside of the container to remove any liquid gasoline or gasoline residue.
- Secure the container in the trunk or pickup so turns or road vibrations won't cause it to slide around or tip over.

- Do not leave a container of gasoline in direct sun, or in the trunk of a car that is in direct sun. Heating the gasoline will build up pressure in the container.
- Never store the gasoline container next to the termite rig pump motor.
- When fueling equipment, wipe up any spills immediately and move the equipment at least 10 feet away from the fueling area to start the engine. Before refueling, turn off the equipment and let it cool completely.

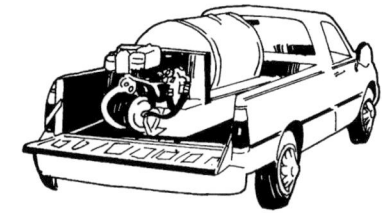

Never store a gasoline container next to the termite rig pump motor

PCBs

Electrical transformers and other devices used to be made with PCBs— polychlorinated biphenyls. These chemical compounds were found to pose environmental and health risks, and their use has been discontinued. Old equipment may still contain PCBs, however, and technicians are at some risk of exposure when working in electrical vaults and around large transformers. Check warning signs before entering electrical vaults. If you find liquid leaking in electrical vaults, stop work and notify the site manager and your supervisor. If you service electrical vaults regularly, do not wear your work shoes when at home or you might track PCBs inside.

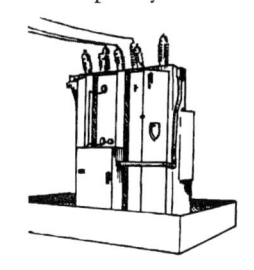

Old transformers may leak dangerous PCBs

Pesticides and Terrorism

Keeping pesticides safely stored and out of the hands of the general public has always been a concern of the pest control industry. Now, the U.S. Department of Homeland Security is worried about pesticides and application equipment getting into the hands of terrorists.

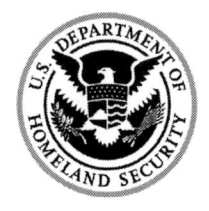

It is up to your company to handle most of the security issues such as making sure the storage site is secure and that pesticides are regularly inventoried. But, some of the security concerns must be handled at the technician level as well.

- Help insure that your company's pesticide storage area remains locked and secure. Only employees and authorized persons are allowed access to the storage area.
- Make sure that your truck or pest control vehicle is kept locked at all times. Never leave ignition keys in vehicles.
- Never leave your service kit, pesticides, or equipment sitting in the hallway while you service an apartment or office.
- Any pesticides marked for disposal should be kept in a locked storage area until they are disposed of.
- Never sell or give pesticides to anyone that is not a known customer.
- Application equipment such as sprayers, tanks, and pumps should be locked up when not in use.
- Report any missing pesticides or equipment to your supervisor immediately.
- Report any suspicious persons or activity around your office or work site.

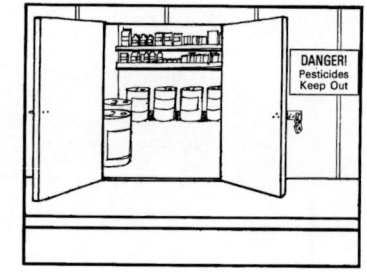

Make sure that pesticide storage areas remain locked and secure.

Key Points to Remember—Pesticides & Chemicals

- √ **Because you use them every day, <u>you</u> are the person most at risk from pesticides.**
- √ **OSHA's Hazard Communication Standard is a set of rules that your company must follow so that you get the information you need to protect yourself from pesticides and other hazardous chemicals.**
- √ **The MSDS is your guide to the potential hazards of a pesticide or other chemical.**
- √ **A signal word (DANGER, WARNING, or CAUTION) is printed on a pesticide label to show you how toxic the product is.**
- √ **Skin absorption is faster with emulsifiable concentrates, as a rule, than with wettable powders or dry formulations.**

- √ **The primary risk to applicators from dust formulations is inhaling the dust while filling equipment and during application.**
- √ **Gasoline is a hazardous chemical both because it is extremely flammable and because you can get sick or injured from breathing its vapors, swallowing it, or spilling it on yourself.**
- √ **For security's sake, keep tight control on your pesticides and application equipment.**

PESTICIDE POISONING

Most of the pesticides you work with have relatively low toxicity to humans. But even with these pesticides, overexposure can cause injury, especially when mixing concentrates. Exposure can occur through the skin (dermal), mouth (oral), lungs (inhalation), or through the eyes. You should know the symptoms of pesticide poisoning in yourself and you should know how to recognize signs of poisoning in coworkers and others who may have been overexposed.

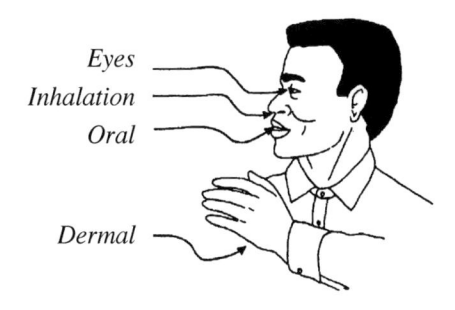

Pesticides can enter the body in four ways

Many of the signs and symptoms of pesticide poisoning are similar to other illnesses which you might experience, such as the flu or even a hangover. A bad headache or nausea may or may not be a warning sign of poisoning. Generally you will have three or more of these early symptoms if you have been poisoned with a pesticide:

- skin irritation
- soreness in joints
- fatigue and weakness
- blurred vision
- moodiness
- nausea
- loss of appetite
- irritation of nose and throat
- eye irritation
- headache
- dizziness
- restlessness
- sweating
- diarrhea or cramps
- thirst
- "pinpoint" pupils

If you, a coworker, or a customer have been in a situation in which pesticide overexposure could occur and you notice suspicious symptoms, first stop the exposure. Speed is essential. Step one in first aid treatment is to prevent absorption of the pesticide.

Remove the individual from the pesticide (get away from the vicinity) or remove the pesticide from the individual (wash it off). Then get medical attention as soon as possible. Provide details on the pesticide involved.

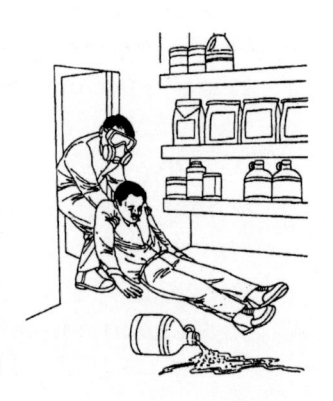

The first step is to stop further exposure to the pesticide

Skin (Dermal) Exposure

Ninety-seven percent of all pesticide exposure during spraying is by contact with the skin. Some pesticide formulations are absorbed through skin more readily than others. Emulsifiable concentrates and oil-based sprays are the most absorptive through skin. Dusts and granules are the least absorptive, and water-based sprays such as wettable powders are somewhere in the middle. Health risks from skin exposure are obviously higher when skin is exposed to a pesticide concentrate rather than a dilution.

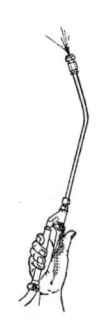

A leaky spray wand can drip insecticide down your arm

The area of the body exposed and the condition of the skin will make a difference in the amount of pesticide absorbed. The genital area, the scalp, ear canal and forehead absorb pesticide very rapidly. Cuts, scrapes, and skin rashes absorb pesticide more quickly than unbroken skin. Hot, sweaty skin also absorbs more pesticide than cool, dry skin.

One common problem is application above eye level with a compressed air sprayer. With the wand held towards the ceiling, the insecticide can drip back down the handle onto the technician's hand. The problem is made worse if the sprayer has a leaky valve or if the insecticide is applied at high pressure. If this skin exposure is repeated day after day, there is a definite health risk.

Causes of Skin Exposure

Skin exposure can be caused by: (1) splashing, dripping, or spraying pesticides on unprotected skin; (2) wearing inadequate personal protective equipment or wearing clothing, gloves, or shoes that are already contaminated with pesticide; (3) applying pesticides outdoors in windy weather; (4) touching pesticide-treated surfaces; and (5) not washing hands after handling pesticides or pesticide containers.

Label Precautions

Before handling a pesticide, look for a *Precautionary Statement* on the label that will alert you to the need for skin protection: "Harmful if absorbed through skin," or "May be a skin sensitizer." The label may specify the use of gloves and wearing long sleeves, in addition to other precautions.

Symptoms of Skin Exposure

Contact with some pesticides can cause your skin to itch, blister, crack, or change color. Extreme skin exposure, particularly to concentrates, can progress to nausea, cramps, sweating, difficulty breathing and other more serious symptoms. Continued skin exposure to some pesticides over a period of time can cause delayed health effects. Some pyrethroids may cause a mild and temporary skin sensitization (see below) or allergic type skin reaction in some individuals.

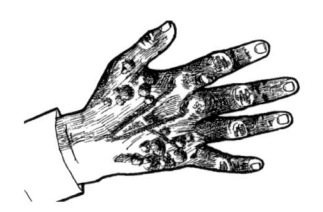

Some pesticides can cause your skin to itch, blister, crack, or change color

First Aid for Pesticide on the Skin

Follow label directions for first aid. If label directions are unavailable, do the following:

(1) *Immediately* drench the skin and clothing with plenty of cool water.
(2) Remove contaminated clothing, jewelry, and equipment.
(3) Wash exposed skin and hair with soap and water.
(4) Cover any burns with clean cloths or bandages. Don't apply any first aid ointments.
(5) For burns or after exposure to highly toxic concentrates, see a physician and bring the pesticide label and MSDS.
(6) Also see a physician if any symptoms persist.

Pyrethroid Skin Sensation

Pyrethroid insecticides can cause a tingling or burning sensation (not an actual burn) and numbness in exposed skin of sensitive people. The symptoms usually appear within two hours of contact with skin and can last up to 24 hours. The degree of skin sensation produced from least to most irritating appears to be as follows: bifenthrin (rare), permethrin (rare), cyfluthrin, cypermethrin, cyhalothrin, deltamethrin, and fenvalerate. Pyrethroid skin sensation is dependent on the formulation, amount of exposure, and a person's sensitivity to a particular product.

Wash your skin with soap and water, and apply an oil-based skin cream to reduce the burning sensation.

Most pyrethroids are low-hazard insecticides. Nevertheless, for your own health and safety, avoid skin contact and protect your eyes. And never expose yourself to *any* insecticide repeatedly or over a long period of time without adequate protection.

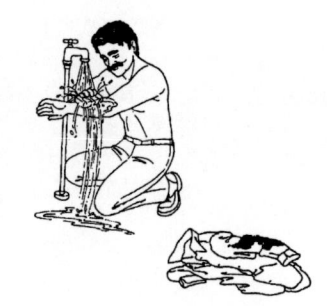

If a pesticide gets on you, strip off contaminated clothes, jewelry, and PPE and wash thoroughly

Oral Exposure

You may think there's no way you could ever swallow pesticide. But oral exposure to pesticide can occur in less obvious ways, for example when you have pesticide on your hands and then chew your fingernails, smoke a cigarette, or eat a sandwich. Or, you might absentmindedly blow into a nozzle or hose to clear it.

Besides the potential for poisoning yourself by mouth, you need to be aware of the potential for other people, especially children, to get pesticide on or in their mouths. Don't spray around food or dishes, or children's toys. Pesticide residue on any of these objects can be easily transferred to the mouth. Children may accidentally drink pesticide or swallow bait thinking that it's food.

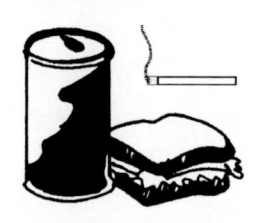

Pesticide residues can be transferred to food, drink, smokes

Causes of Oral Exposure

Oral exposure can be caused by (1) not washing your hands before eating, drinking, smoking, or chewing; (2) accidentally splashing pesticide in your mouth when pouring or applying it; (3) accidentally applying pesticide to food, cigarettes, or other objects that then go into your mouth; (4) wiping your mouth with a contaminated hand; and (5) mistaking pesticide for food or drink.

Label Precautions

Before using a pesticide, look for a *Precautionary Statement* on the label that will alert you to the degree of oral hazard: "May be harmful if swallowed" for a pesticide with a slight oral toxicity, or "Fatal if swallowed" or "Can kill you if swallowed" for a highly toxic pesticide.

Symptoms of Oral Exposure

Oral exposure to certain pesticides can burn your mouth or throat and make it difficult to swallow. Some pesticides that are swallowed can burn your digestive system. Others won't cause any acute burning symptoms but can be carried through your blood stream and cause various chronic or delayed health effects. For some restricted-use pesticides, swallowing even a few drops from a splash or wiping your mouth with a contaminated glove can make you very ill.

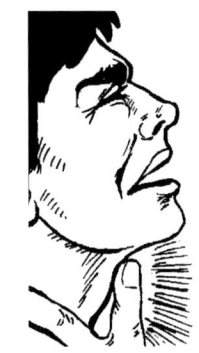

Oral exposure to some pesticides can burn your mouth or throat

First Aid for Swallowed Pesticide

It's particularly important to read the pesticide label's directions for oral poisoning since the first aid procedures are not the same for all types of pesticides. If the label is not available:

(1) Rinse your mouth with plenty of water.
(2) Drink large amounts (up to 1 quart) of milk or water.
(3) Induce vomiting only if the pesticide label, manufacturer, or poison control expert advises you to do so. In general, vomiting should <u>not</u> be induced if you are having convulsions, or if you have swallowed an emulsifiable concentrate or oil solution, or a strong acid or alkali poison.
(4) Get to a physician as soon as possible.

Inhalation Exposure

Inhalation of a pesticide simply means that the pesticide has been breathed in. How this will affect you depends on the toxicity of the pesticide, how much you have inhaled, and how long you have been breathing it. You can be poisoned by inhaling any airborne pesticide: aerosols, liquid sprays, fumigant gases, or dusts.

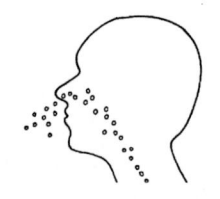

Inhalation exposure is a special hazard in crawlspaces and other enclosed areas

Inhalation can be a hazard if you are working in a poorly-ventilated, enclosed space like a crawlspace, attic, or manhole. Fumigators need to be especially careful to avoid inhaling a fumigant which can be fatal.

Causes of Inhalation Exposure

Inhalation exposure can be caused by: (1) failing to use the proper respirator when necessary; (2) using a respirator that doesn't fit properly or using old or inadequate filters, cartridges, or canisters; (3) using pesticides in closed or poorly-ventilated spaces and not wearing a respirator; (4) spills and improper storage in storage facility or vehicle; (5) inhaling vapors or dusts after application, for example reentering an area too soon; or (6) inhaling pesticide drift from a treated area.

Label Precautions

Before handling a pesticide, look for a *Precautionary Statement* on the label that will alert you to an inhalation hazard: "Harmful if inhaled," or "Do not breathe dusts, vapors, or spray mist," or "Inhalation may cause delayed lung, nerve, or brain injury." The label may specify the use of a specific type or model of respirator.

Symptoms of Inhalation Exposure

Some inhaled pesticides may cause *acute* or immediate effects. They may "burn" your respiratory system, making it difficult to breathe. Other pesticides may not affect your breathing at all but may be carried through your blood stream causing other harmful effects. You may develop flu-like symptoms such as nausea, headache, chills, and aches. In some cases, the effects of inhaling a pesticide may result in delayed, or *chronic*, effects that appear days later. Continuous or frequent inhalation exposure to some pesticides over a long period of time can result in emphysema or asthma that appears years later.

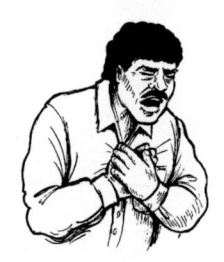

Some inhaled pesticides cause acute lung pain, others cause chronic effects days later

> *First Aid for Inhaled Pesticide*
>
> If someone needs first aid after inhaling a pesticide, do the following:
>
> (1) Get the victim away from the pesticide vapors and into fresh air immediately.
> (2) If other people are in the same area, warn them of the danger.
> (3) Loosen any tight clothing on the victim.
> (4) If the victim has stopped breathing, immediately call 911 (if possible) and administer CPR.
> (5) Keep the victim warm and quiet.
> (6) Get the victim to a hospital or physician.
> (7) Take the pesticide container, label, and MSDS with you.

Eye Exposure

The health effects from pesticide exposure to an eye depend on the toxicity of the pesticide, how much pesticide is involved, and how long the pesticide remains in contact with the eye. The effects can range from simple eye irritation to eye burns to permanent blindness from some highly corrosive pesticides. Some pesticides may not irritate your eyes at all but can pass through your eyes and enter your body causing internal poisoning. The eyes offer a very fast route for pesticide absorption.

Causes of Eye Exposure

You can get pesticide in your eyes by: (1) accidentally splashing or spraying pesticides into your eyes; (2) applying pesticides in windy conditions without eye protection; (3) rubbing your eyes with contaminated gloves or hands; or (4) having dusts, wettable powders, or granules drift into unprotected eyes.

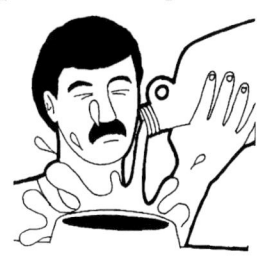

Watch out for splashing pesticide concentrate

Label Precautions

Before handling a pesticide, look for a *Precautionary Statement* on the label that will alert you to the need for eye protection: "Avoid contact with eyes," or "May irritate eyes," or "Causes eye burns." The label may specify the use of a specific type of safety eyewear, such as goggles, at least when pouring or mixing the product.

Pest Control Technician Safety Manual

Symptoms of Eye Exposure

Usually you will know right away if you have gotten pesticide in your eyes. The acute symptoms that occur immediately may include burning or tearing. Even if there is no irritation, you must take immediate first aid measures to keep the pesticide from entering your system.

First Aid for Pesticide in the Eyes

Wash the eye or eyes quickly, but gently. Follow these procedures:

(1) Use an eye wash dispenser if available (see discussion of eye protection under *Pesticide PPE*). Otherwise, use a garden hose or faucet.
(2) Hold the eye open and wash with a gentle flow of water across the eye. Continue to rinse the affected eye or eyes for at least 15 minutes.
(3) Don't use eye drops afterwards.
(4) Inform your supervisor.
(5) Check with a physician if advised to do so on the label, or if you have any remaining symptoms (irritation, blurred vision, etc.)

Key Points to Remember—Pesticide Poisoning

- √ **Most pesticide exposure during spraying is by contact with the skin.**
- √ **The genital area, the scalp, eyes, ear canal and forehead absorb pesticide very rapidly.**
- √ **Pyrethroid insecticides can cause a tingling or burning sensation and numbness in exposed skin.**
- √ **Technicians can get pesticides in their mouth by chewing on contaminated fingernails, smoking a cigarette or eating with contaminated hands, or blowing in a nozzle or hose to clear it.**
- √ **Your risk of inhaling a pesticide is higher if you are working in a poorly-ventilated, restricted space like a crawlspace, attic, or manhole.**
- √ **Wash your eye(s) out with water for at least 15 minutes if it is splashed with a pesticide.**

PESTICIDE PPE

PPE is short for personal protective equipment. Some PPE is used to protect you from exposure to pesticides. Examples include chemical-resistant gloves, respirators, even long-sleeved shirts and pants. The PPE you use will depend on the pesticide product (check the label for minimum requirements), the application technique, and specific conditions at the site.

Choosing Protective Equipment

What if the pesticide label says you should wear "protective eyewear" when applying the product? Do your regular glasses count as protective eyewear? Sorry, no. What if the label says wear chemical-resistant gloves? Can you use vinyl dishwashing gloves? Again, no. PPE must be designed to protect you from the particular hazards of the pesticide, or at least have been shown to be sufficient to protect you. See the chart *Choosing Pesticide PPE* on the next page to help determine what qualifies as adequate personal protective equipment. The labeling statement is for the minimum level of protection required. You can always choose PPE that provides a larger measure of safety.

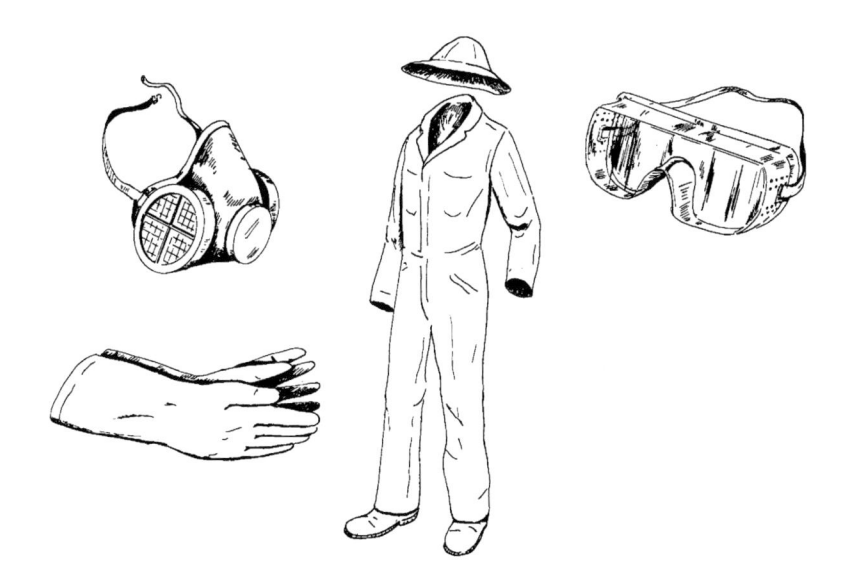

Required PPE can include respirator, gloves, hat, coveralls, and eye protection. Follow the label

Pest Control Technician Safety Manual

Choosing Pesticide PPE

IF THE LABEL REQUIRES...	WEAR ANY ONE OF THESE...
protective eyewear	(1) shielded safety glasses (2) goggles (3) face shield (4) full-face style respirator
goggles	(1) goggles (2) full-face style respirator
dust/mist filtering respirator	(1) dust/mist respirator (2) respirator w/ dust/mist filtering cartridge (3) respirator w/ organic vapor-removing cartridge and pesticide prefilter (4) respirator w/ canister approved for pesticides (5) air-supplying respirator
cartridge respirator	(1) respirator w/ organic vapor-removing cartridge and pesticide prefilter (2) respirator w/ canister approved for pesticides (3) air-supplying respirator
long-sleeved shirt and long-legged pants	(1) long-sleeved shirt and pants (2) woven or nonwoven coveralls (3) plastic or coated coveralls (4) rubber or plastic suit
waterproof gloves	(1) sturdy rubber or plastic gloves
chemical-resistant gloves	(1) barrier laminate gloves (2) gloves that the manufacturer indicates are chemically-resistant to the pesticide
chemical-resistant gloves such as butyl or nitrile	(1) butyl gloves (2) nitrile gloves (3) gloves that the manufacturer indicates are chemically-resistant to the pesticide
chemical-resistant footwear	(1) chemical-resistant shoes (2) chemical-resistant boots (3) chemical-resistant booties or shoe coverings

Respirators

Respirators have to be worn whenever airborne contaminants may affect your health and safety. Most pest control technicians wear a respirator at least some of the time when mixing or applying pesticides. OSHA requires that pest control companies have a *Respiratory Protective Program* in place. As part of the program, you receive a medical evaluation to determine that you can use a respirator, and instruction in selecting, fitting, inspecting, maintaining, cleaning, storing, and using your respirator.

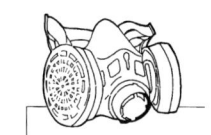

Respirators must be worn if you face an airborne hazard

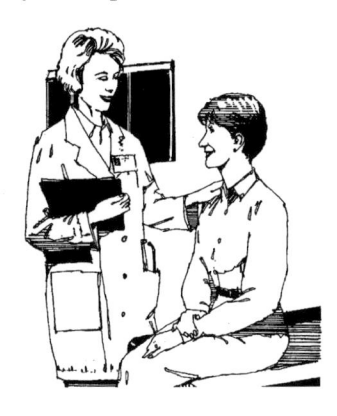

Any worker using a respirator MUST have a medical evaluation

Medical Evaluation

Using a respirator stresses your body because breathing is restricted. How much stress depends on the type of respirator, job conditions, and your health. Certain medical conditions, such as heart or lung trouble, affect your ability to use a respirator safely. Other factors that affect your ability to use a respirator safely include beards, dentures, the shape of your face, some types of glasses, and the use of certain medications. OSHA rules require that all workers using a respirator undergo a medical evaluation, either a medical questionnaire or a physical exam, to determine if they are medically and physically able to use a respirator.

Selection and Fit

Your respirator must be suited to the particular hazards you face, and it must fit properly in order to work. The first step in respirator training is selection of the proper type and size of respirator for the individual and the job. Most technicians use a cartridge respirator, but technicians doing fumigation may need a self-contained breathing apparatus (SCBA), and technicians who wear glasses may need a full facepiece respirator to get an adequate seal. Make sure your respirators and cartridges are NIOSH-approved. (NIOSH, the National Institute of Occupational Safety and Health, tests and certifies safety equipment.)

    Cartridge respirators come in different sizes and styles. You need to find the one that will seal completely on your face when adjusted. No air should escape around the edges of the facepiece. (Beards make a tight seal difficult and sometimes impossible.) A *fit test* will determine if your respirator fits properly. There are different ways to do a fit test. A sophisticated fit test chamber can measure the presence of an aerosol inside and outside of the respirator facepiece. But most pest control companies use a simple substance detection test to check the fit. For example, an odor test uses banana oil; a taste test uses saccharin; other tests use a harmless irritant or smoke. They all work the same way. While you wear your selected respirator, the substance is wafted into the air in front of you. If you can smell it, taste it, or otherwise detect it, your respirator doesn't fit properly.

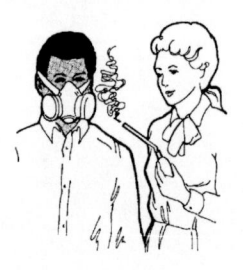

A respirator must fit correctly in order to protect you

Once you've found a respirator that fits, you must repeat the fit test every year...or more often, if you gain or lose weight, or get dentures or glasses.

Check the condition of your respirator each time you wear it, and conduct a "user seal check" to recheck the fit. It only takes a few seconds. Seal checks can be *positive pressure tests* or *negative pressure tests*. For positive pressure tests, cover the exhalation valve with your hand (you may have to first remove the valve cover). Press lightly and exhale gently. If the fit is correct, you should feel the facepiece bulge slightly from trapped air. If air is escaping, recheck and refit.

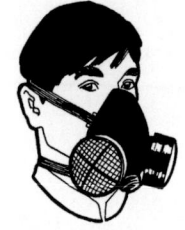

Do a seal check each time you use your respirator

For a negative pressure test, close off the inlet openings by covering them with the palms of your hands, or by replacing the filter seals. Then inhale gently so that the facepiece collapses slightly, and hold your breath for ten seconds. If the facepiece stays collapsed, and no air is leaking, the fit is correct.

Inspection and Maintenance

You need to know how to inspect and maintain your respirators. According to OSHA, *all respirators must be inspected for wear and deterioration...before and after each use.* Special attention should be given to the rubber or plastic parts which can crack or lose flexibility.

The following maintenance steps are for a cartridge respirator. Full facepiece and air-supplying respirators will require additional inspection.

(1) Check the **facepiece** for dirt and grime, cracks, or tears. Make sure the shape of the facepiece is not distorted from improper storage or from deterioration of the material.
(2) Check the **headstraps** for cracking, loss of elasticity, or broken buckles or attachments.
(3) Remove the cover of the **exhalation valve** and check for dirt, debris, or hairs under the valve seat. Look for cracks or tears in the valve material and cracks or chips in the valve body. Make sure the valve is seated properly in the valve body.
(4) Check the **cartridges**. Look for improper installation, loose connections, missing or worn gaskets. Check for cracks or dents in the outside case of the cartridge. Make sure you are using a cartridge and filter that are approved by NIOSH/MSHA for the pesticides you apply. Check the shelf-life date on the cartridge.

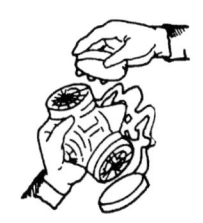

Check the valves and cartridges for damage and debris

While you're examining your respirator, stretch and work the rubber parts to restore pliability and prevent warping or sticking during storage.

Follow the respirator manufacturer's guidelines for repairs or replacement of parts. Repairs should be made only by trained persons using parts supplied by the manufacturer that are specific for the make and model of the respirator.

Replacing Respirator Cartridges and Filters

Respirators designed to protect you from pesticide dusts, mists, and vapors use a cartridge filtration system. A chemical cartridge is a container filled with a sorbent material (usually activated charcoal) which absorbs the vapor molecules in the air before you inhale them. Most also use a pre-filter.

Cartridges and filters gradually lose their protective ability. *Most technicians don't change cartridges and filters often enough.*

When should you replace respirator cartridges and filters? The useful life of respirator filters and cartridges depends on (1) the amount of particles in the air, (2) the concentration of vapor being filtered, (3) the amount of absorbent material that they contain, (4) the breathing rate of the wearer, (5) the temperature and humidity, and (6) the length of time that they've been stored between uses.

When a respirator cartridge has absorbed as much of the airborne vapors as it can, the vapors will begin to pass through the cartridge and enter the facepiece. That's not good!

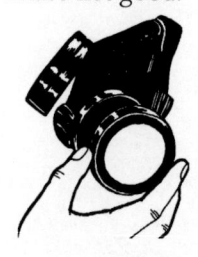

Change cartridges according to your employer's cartridge change-out schedule or the respirator manufacturer's guidelines. Using a change-out schedule means you should be replacing cartridges before you notice any problem. The cartridge replacement period has to be based on the most volatile chemical that you are exposed to in your work.

Change cartridges as specified or if you have a "breakthrough"

If there are no guidelines or formal schedule, change cartridges after about 8 hours of use or any time you experience "breakthrough"...in other words if you smell pesticides or have dizziness or trouble breathing.

Respirator particulate filters or pre-filters typically need changing more often than cartridges in dusty environments. Change respirator filters twice a day or even more often under heavy usage or if breathing becomes difficult.

There are several types of respirator cartridges to remove specific vapors and gases. Make sure you are using a cartridge and filter that are approved by NIOSH/MSHA for the pesticides you apply. If you have a reusable cartridge respirator, you can change cartridges when you face different types of contaminants. However, do not interchange cartridges from different manufacturers; different threading won't allow a proper fit. Check the shelf-life date on the cartridge.

Cleaning Your Respirator

Respirators need to be cleaned and disinfected frequently. If a respirator is shared with another worker, it must be cleaned and disinfected after <u>each</u> use.

(1) Handle the respirator only with clean hands and use only clean drying cloths that have not been contaminated with pesticides.

(2) Remove filters and cartridges.

(3) Wash the facepiece according to manufacturer's guidelines, or use a mix of detergent, bleach, and warm water, or a commercially-available cleaner and dis-infectant solution. Do not use ammonia, hot water, or strong cleaning detergents or chemicals as they can damage respirator parts.

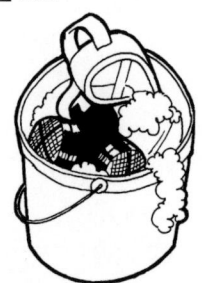

Wash the facepiece in warm water with mild detergent and bleach

(4) Rinse the respirator <u>thoroughly</u> in warm water, preferably running water, and wipe dry with a clean lint-free cloth, or hang to air dry.

(5) Reassemble and test to make sure the respirator works and seals properly.

(Note: A respirator that has been contaminated with a concentrated pesticide may require a separate decontamination procedure. In such a case, check with the manufacturer of your respirator.)

Storing Your Respirator

After cleaning and drying, seal the entire respirator in a sturdy, airtight container like a zip-lock plastic bag. OSHA requires that respirators *be stored in a convenient, clean, and sanitary location.* Store respirators where they're protected from dust, sunlight, extreme temperatures, moisture, pesticides, and other chemicals. Store respirators so that they sit in a normal position to prevent distortion of the shape of the rubber or plastic parts.

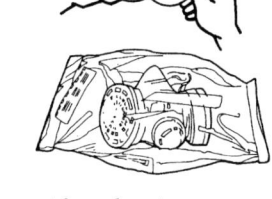

After cleaning, store your respirator in an airtight container such as a plastic bag

During the work day, respirators stored in your vehicle should be kept away from pesticides. Don't throw your respirator into a service kit or locker unless it is protected in a carrying case or box.

High Efficiency (HE) Respirators and Filters

When you work around rodent or bird droppings, asbestos, or in certain medical facilities, you often need to wear a respirator equipped with a high efficiency filter that is at least 99.97% efficient in removing...particles of 0.3 micrometers in diameter. Such filters used to be designated HEPA filters (for High Efficiency Particulate Air filter). The HEPA designation has been replaced by a new class of filters.

The National Institute of Occupational Safety and Health (NIOSH) is the government group responsible for testing and rating respirators and other safety equipment. NIOSH has upgraded the respirator standard to improve respirator resistance to oil and to better remove small particles such as mold spores or silica.

The old HEPA filters have been replaced by N-100, R-100, and P-100 filters and respirators. The new type 100s are instead designated "HE" (high efficiency). They are at least 99.97% efficient in filtering particles down to the 0.3 micron range, and are equivalent to the old HEPA filter. The cartridges are the same purple color as the older HEPA filter but are smaller in size.

If your work calls for a HEPA-type filter, make sure you use a 100 series respirator, cartridge, or filter. There are also 95 and 99 series filters but these will not give you the high level of protection needed. Older HEPA filters can be used until the supply runs out.

In the new filter designation, "N" filters are not resistant to oil or solvent, "R" filters are oil and solvent-resistant for 8 hours, and "P" filters are oil and solvent-proof. For work around animal droppings or asbestos, an N-100 filter would suffice.

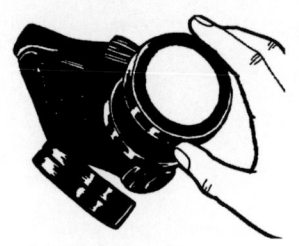

The Centers for Disease Control states that the N-100 filter should provide the same protection as the HEPA filter against hantavirus. An N-100 filter is suitable for protecting against extremely fine and very toxic particles when there is no oil or solvent in the air. If there is also oil or solvent in the air, you should choose a R-100 or P-100 filter. If you're exposed to organic vapors, make sure the filter is also rated for organic vapors.

A 100 series filter protects against all particulates including viruses

A 100 series filter will protect you against all particulates including viruses, bacteria, and other microorganisms, fecal and urinary particles, asbestos or fiberglass, animal or insect dander and allergens. But it's important to have the right respirator fit. Even a 100 series filter won't protect you from viral or asbestos particles if a poor seal allows air to bypass the filter in your respirator. You should conduct a fit test with the same make, model, style, and size of respirator that you will be using.

Gloves

When mixing or applying pesticides, most of your exposure is through your hands and forearms. Consequently, many pesticide labels require you to wear chemical-resistant gloves. A glove is considered "chemical-resistant" if there can be no movement of pesticide through the material during its use. Sometimes the label or MSDS will specify what type of gloves are resistant to the pesticide or solvents in the product. The label may tell you to wear "chemical-resistant gloves such as butyl or nitrile." If the label does not specifically advise you, use your own judgement. A rubber glove that qualifies as

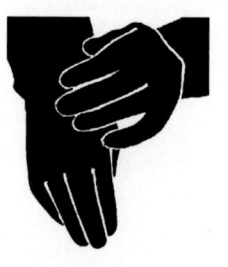

Many pesticides require that you use "chemical-resistant" gloves

chemical-resistant if you're applying a wettable powder may not be considered chemical-resistant if you're using a liquid concentrate.

(Be warned that latex rubber gloves may trigger allergic reactions in some wearers. See *Allergy*.)

EPA Allows the Use of Glove Liners

The Environmental Protection Agency made a change in the Worker Protection Standard that applies to protective gloves. Pesticide applicators can now wear separate glove liners underneath chemical-resistant gloves when those gloves are required for pesticide mixing or application.

The glove liners may not be longer than the chemical-resistant glove and they may not extend outside the glove. The liners must be disposed of after 10 hours of use or whenever the liners become contaminated.

EPA took this action to reduce the discomfort of unlined chemical-resistant gloves, especially during very hot or cold weather. Lined or flocked gloves, where the lining is attached to the inside of the chemical-resistant outer glove, remain unacceptable because pesticide can soak into the lining resulting in continuous exposure for the wearer.

Guidelines for Dry Pesticides or Water-based Pesticides

Dry pesticides are dusts, granules, pellets, and most baits. Water-based pesticides include wettable powders, soluble powders, some solutions, microencapsulates, and dry flowables. If you are handling or applying any of these formulations, *any thick plastic or rubber glove* is considered chemical-resistant as long as it is unlined and has sealed seams.

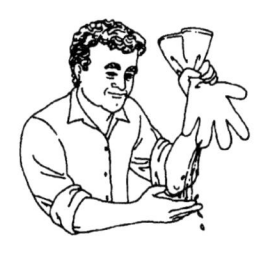

Water can be used to check gloves for leaks

Gloves made of absorbent material like cotton, leather, or canvas are not chemical-resistant even to dry formulations. They are impossible to clean thoroughly and should never be worn when handling pesticides (except in the case of certain fumigants, which require the use of cotton gloves).

Guidelines for Non-water-based Liquid Pesticides

Liquid pesticides that are not water-based include emulsifiable concentrates, ultra-low-volume and low-volume concentrates, flowables, aerosols, and invert emulsions. These formulations usually contain solvents like xylene, petroleum distillates, or alcohol. Your choice of a chemical-resistant glove depends on the solvent used which may or may not be listed on the product label. If you are handling or applying a formulation that contains a solvent, choose *gloves made of butyl, nitrile, or foil-laminate*, or as indicated by label instructions.

Guidelines for Fumigants

Follow the label instructions regarding gloves precisely. Some fumigants specifically warn you NOT to wear waterproof or rubber gloves because they can trap the fumigant gas against your skin and cause severe burns and absorption. Some fumigants require that you use cotton gloves.

Eye Protection

Pest control technicians often need eye protection when using pesticides. Pesticide can splash into your eyes when pouring, or it can splash back during application. You may need eye protection from airborne pesticides when applying certain aerosol, dust, or space treatments.

Always check the pesticide label to see what type of safety eyewear is required. If the label simply says, "Avoid getting in eyes," that should be a hint to you to wear protective eyewear at least when you are pouring or mixing the product. The type of eye protection you choose must:

- provide adequate protection against the particular hazards (such as chemical splash) you are facing
- be reasonably comfortable when worn under work conditions
- fit snugly, without interfering with your movements or vision
- be durable
- be capable of being disinfected and be easily cleanable
- be kept clean and in good repair

Regular glasses do not provide enough eye protection

If you wear prescription eyeglasses and you are required to wear eye protection on the job, your regular glasses are not enough. You must wear prescription shielded safety glasses, prescription goggles, goggles over your prescription glasses, a face shield, or a full facepiece respirator.

Inspect and clean protective eyewear daily. Replace pitted or badly scratched lenses. Replace headbands that are worn and no longer have the elasticity to hold the goggles in place. Safety eyewear that is worn by more than one employee needs to be disinfected after each use. Store safety glasses or goggles in a clean, dust-proof case, box, or zip-closing plastic bag.

Changing Views on Contact Lenses and Pesticides

Some pest control companies and many safety experts discouraged or prohibited wearing contact lenses during pesticide application. The reason? Contact lenses were thought to trap contaminants, such as pesticides, against the eye underneath the lenses.

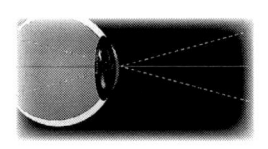

No additional hazards to contact lens wearers

Photo © Royce DeGrie/iStockphoto

Safety experts are changing their opinions on the issue of contact lenses and eye hazards. Recent studies have shown no additional hazards to contact lens wearers during chemical exposures, and have even suggested that contact lenses help protect the eye from immediate, direct contact with the highest concentration of a hazardous substance.

The American Chemical Society's (ACS) Committee on Chemical Safety believes that "contact lenses can actually minimize and prevent injuries in many situations." The American Optometric Association (AOA) agrees, stating that "some types of contact lenses may give added protection...in instances of certain fume exposure, chemical splash, dust, flying particles, and optical radiation."

OSHA believes that contact lenses do not pose additional hazards to the wearer, and has determined that "additional regulation addressing the use of contact lenses is unnecessary." OSHA warns, however, that "contact lenses are not eye protective devices. If eye hazards are present, appropriate eye protection must be worn instead of, or in conjunction with, contact lenses."

What do these changes mean to technicians? Absent any scientific data demonstrating that there are special hazards from using contact lenses around pesticides, it will not be necessary for technicians to remove contact lenses when there are eye hazards, as long as proper eye protection (goggle, shield, etc.) is worn.

However, if the pesticide label or supporting labeling prohibit contact lens use, then applicators should not wear them. *Label directions and precautions always take precedence over suggestions or other guidelines.*

What Kind of Eye Protection Is Best?

Under the *Precautionary Statements* section, the pesticide label often states, "wear safety glasses, goggles, or face shield when handling undiluted material." Which is your best choice for protective eyewear?

As mentioned earlier, regular prescription eyeglasses do not qualify as protective eyewear. Pesticide can still splash in from the sides. Contact lenses definitely do not qualify. Protective eyewear must be made of chemical-resistant plastic and must shield your eyes on all sides.

Goggles—This is the protective eyewear most often used by pest control technicians. Goggles fit tightly against the face and protect the eyes from all sides, yet they are easy to carry and use. Some styles are designed to be worn over eyeglasses. Most can be worn with half-face respirators. Goggles can be vented at the sides, or not. Unvented goggles are preferred when applying mists, fogs, or aerosols.

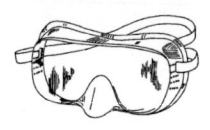

Vented goggles are less likely to fog, but aerosols and mists may get inside

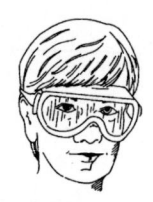

Unvented goggles protect your eyes when applying any pesticide

Shielded Safety Glasses—Safety glasses provide protection in many situations. They are comfortable, less apt to "fog" up than other protective eyewear, and can be worn with a half-face respirator. Safety glasses must have attached brow and side panels.

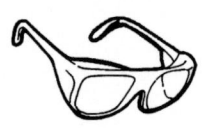

Safety glasses must have attached brow and side panels

Face shields protect against splashback and can be worn with eyeglasses

Face Shields—Because they have the added benefit of protecting your entire face from pesticide splashes, face shields are especially useful during mixing. They may be the best choice for people who must wear prescription eyeglasses since they don't fit tightly against the temples.

Emergency Eye Washes

Pest control technicians are required by the pesticide label and by OSHA to wear protective goggles or other eyewear when handling or applying certain pesticides. Regardless, accidents happen. Pesticides or solvents can splash or blow into your eyes during pouring, mixing, or applying.

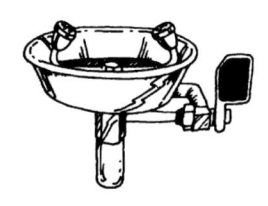

Chemicals can scar or burn your eyes, permanently affecting vision. Your eyes are also a direct route for poison to enter the body (see discussion of eye exposure under *Pesticide Poisoning*). It's important that any liquid chemical splashed into your eyes be flushed out immediately and thoroughly. There are various types of eyewash devices specifically designed to do this, such as installed eyewash fountains, faucet-mounted emergency eye wash stations, and portable eye wash devices. Here are some guidelines for flushing chemicals from your eyes:

If pesticide splashes in your eyes, flush them immediately with water

- To correctly use an eyewash, the upper and lower eyelids must be held wide apart with your fingers. Flush a continuous stream of cool, clean water upward across the eye for at least 15 minutes. Blink and roll your eye as much as possible so that the water reaches all parts of the eye. Don't use eye drops in place of flushing or after flushing.
- If chemicals splash in your eyes and you are wearing contact lenses, begin flushing the eyes with the contacts still in place. Then remove the contacts and continue flushing.
- If you're on the job and there is no eyewash nearby, use a garden hose to flush your eyes.
- Have your eyes checked by a physician or other medical practitioner.

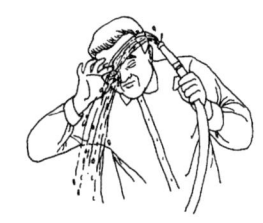

If eyewash equipment is not available, flush your eyes for 15 minutes with a hose or faucet

Clothing

Your regular work clothing is a type of PPE since in some sense and to some degree it keeps pesticide from contacting your skin. Coveralls worn over regular clothing provide additional protection and can be quickly removed if contaminated. Other types of clothing are specifically designed to protect against skin exposure to chemicals.

Pesticides and Fabrics

Research has shown that some clothing fabrics protect you from pesticide spills better than others. It has to do with two characteristics of fabric: absorbency and wicking. Absorbency is the amount of fluid a fabric will soak up and hold. Wicking is the tendency of a fluid to be pulled through the fabric onto underclothes or skin. The chart below summarizes the results.

Absorbancy and Wicking of Various Materials

Material	Absorbency	Wicking
100% Cotton	high	low
Synthetics (nylon, acrylic, polyester)	low	high
Cotton/polyester blends	moderate	moderate
Broadcloth	moderate	high
Spun-bonded olefin (Tyvek®)	low	low

The study found that spun-bonded olefin (DuPont's Tyvek®) offered the greatest level of protection from pesticide. Because standard Tyvek doesn't "breathe", it can be hot to wear, but you should consider disposable Tyvek coveralls over your regular work clothes when you need a high level of protection.

Clothing Treatment

When you're spraying, most of the pesticide that is absorbed into your clothing is from the knees down. You can reduce this by spraying your uniform or pants with Scotchgard™ or a similar fabric protectant. It only costs pennies per treatment and you can wash your pants three times before you need to re-apply it. Scotchgard will reduce by more than 90% the amount of pesticide absorbed by your clothes.

Another protective option, discovered by Cornell University researchers, is ordinary fabric starch sprayed on work clothes. The starch acts as a "pesticide trap," binding with pesticides and keeping them on the clothing and away from the skin. And because the pesticides are bound to the starch, they are more easily removed with the starch during washing.

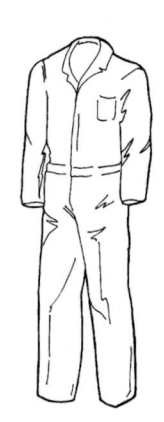

Tyvek suits or coveralls treated with starch will keep pesticide off your skin

Laundry starch adheres well to cotton and cotton/polyester clothing. It's inexpensive, biodegradable, and familiar to most people. And it can be selectively applied to certain areas of clothing that need protection. Starch can also make work clothes more comfortable because it makes them more "breathable," allowing moisture to escape from the skin. Because the protective starch is removed in the wash, it must be reapplied after each laundering.

Washing Work Clothes

The National Institute of Occupational Safety and Health (NIOSH) recently completed a study of home contamination from workers tracking toxic materials home from work. The study showed the workers' families can be inadvertently exposed to hazardous materials unless certain precautions are taken. These precautions include: (1) changing clothes and showering before going home, (2) leaving soiled clothing at work to be laundered by the employer, and (3) storing street clothes in separate areas of the workplace to prevent their contamination. NIOSH also found that normal laundry practices were usually inadequate for cleaning clothing heavily contaminated with toxic materials.

University and government research has led to guidelines for washing pesticide-contaminated work clothes.

- The more "contaminated" the work clothes are, the more thorough the washing should be. Clothes that are saturated with a highly toxic pesticide should be discarded.
- Wash work clothes as soon as possible after wearing them. Store and wash them separately from other family laundry. Use rubber gloves to handle contaminated clothing.
- Presoak the clothing. Use a prewash additive such as *Era®*, *Shout®*, or *Spray and Wash®*.
- Wash the clothes in a full wash cycle using as much **hot** water as possible. Use a heavy-duty, liquid laundry detergent. Use 1-1/2 times the amount of detergent recommended. For more heavily contaminated clothing, repeat the wash cycle. Rinse the washing machine after use.
- Line-dry the clothing outside if possible. Sunlight helps to break down pesticide residues.

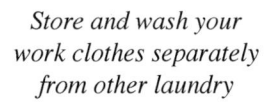

Store and wash your work clothes separately from other laundry

For information on other PPE, see *Noise* (for hearing protectors) and *Head Injury* (for hard hats).

Key Points to Remember—Pesticide PPE

- √ **Respirators MUST be worn whenever airborne contaminants may affect your health and safety.**
- √ **Certain medical conditions, such as heart and lung trouble, can make it unsafe to use a respirator.**
- √ **Check the condition of your respirator each time you wear it, and conduct a seal check to recheck the fit.**
- √ **Store respirators where they are protected from dust, sunlight, extreme temperatures, moisture, pesticides, and other chemicals.**
- √ **When mixing or applying pesticides, most of your exposure is through your hands and forearms.**
- √ **Prescription eyeglasses and contact lenses do not qualify as protective eyewear.**
- √ **Store and wash work clothes separately from other family laundry.**

PETS AND GUARD DOGS

In pest control, you routinely face a risk of being bitten or scratched by pets during residential service, and by guard dogs while servicing commercial accounts after hours.

Pets

Do not trust a customer's assurance that their dog is not going to bite you. Ask them to move the animal to another room or take it out of the residence completely. Do not enter an account with a dog present if no one is home, unless you are sure that the dog poses no threat. Some companies have their technicians carry pepper spray or a similar animal control product in case of attack. Do not touch a dog or cat unless you are sure it is friendly.

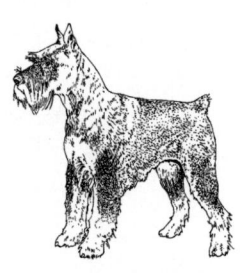

Have pets moved to another room or out of the residence

Guard Dogs

Commercial accounts, such as warehouses, often use trained dogs to guard the grounds during off-hours. Many of these dogs are trained to attack brutally. Periodically ask about guard dogs in each commercial account you service. An account may suddenly begin using a guard dog because of crime in the area, or may change the dog's location or hours. In accounts with a guard dog, do not enter protected areas after hours unless accompanied by an authorized person, or unless you are <u>absolutely</u> sure that no guard dog is loose.

Know What to Do When Confronted by a Dog

Occasionally, on your job, you come in contact with dogs at a customer's house or at a commercial account. What you do when confronted by a dog can determine whether you end up in the emergency room with a severe bite, or not. This is what the experts advise:

- Do not approach strange dogs. Some say you should approach the dog and put your hand out so that it can sniff you. Wrong! It's important that the dog get a sniff, but let the dog approach you; don't approach the dog. This could be perceived as a threat.
- Do not attempt to pet a strange dog until you have completed the sniff test mentioned above, and then only with the owner's permission. If the owner is not available, don't pet the dog. If you do pet a customer's dog, stroke him along the back (which is less threatening) rather than on the head.
- Don't equate a wagging tail with a friendly dog. Tail wagging is a sign of excitement which can be good or bad. A friendly dog wags his tail horizontally or lower than his body and his whole rear end moves. A dog holding his tail high and wagging stiffly is usually a bad sign.

If a dog is threatening, do not make eye contact

- If a dog is threatening, do not make eye contact. Stand tall and still. Do not move until the dog leaves. Never run from a dog since their natural instinct is to chase prey.
- If a dog attacks, try to put an object between you and the dog such as a chair or your sprayer. If you have been knocked to the ground, stay quiet and cover your head with your hands for protection. The dog may see this as a submissive gesture and leave you alone.

Treatment of Bites and Scratches

If you are bitten or scratched by a dog, cat, or other pet, take the following actions:

(1) Get away from the animal and try to confine it to avoid further injury.
(2) Immediately and thoroughly wash the wounds with soap (germicidal, if possible) and water. Allow the wounds to bleed to help deep-cleanse them.
(3) Determine if the animal has been vaccinated for rabies. Do not take the owner's word that the animal has been vaccinated. Obtain a copy of a record of the rabies vaccination for the animal, or the name of the owner's veterinarian. (See also rabies discussion under *Wildlife*.) If you have any problem getting vaccination information, contact your local health department.
(4) See a physician no matter how minor the injury.

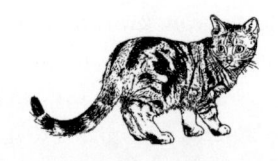

If bitten or scratched, insist on proof that the animal has been vaccinated for rabies

Key Points to Remember—Pets and Guard Dogs

√ **Do not trust a customer's assurance that their dog is not going to bite you.**

√ **Do not enter an account with a dog if no one is at home, unless you are sure that the dog poses no threat.**

√ **Periodically ask about guard dogs in each commercial account you service.**

√ **In accounts with a guard dog, do not enter protected areas after hours unless accompanied by an authorized person, or unless you are <u>absolutely</u> sure that no guard dog is present.**

√ **If a dog is threatening, do not make eye contact.**

√ **If a dog attacks, try to put an object between you and the dog such as a chair or your sprayer.**

√ **If you are bitten or scratched, wash out the wounds, check on the animal's rabies vaccination, and see a physician no matter how minor the injury.**

POISON IVY

An irritating oil in the poison ivy plant (*Rhus radicans*) causes misery for people who touch it (or touch something else that's touched it). It takes the oils only minutes to penetrate the skin but it can take as long as two weeks for allergic reactions to appear. Some people brag that they've never gotten poison ivy. They might be one of the lucky 10-15% of the population that is immune. But most people develop a reaction to it eventually, often after repeated exposures.

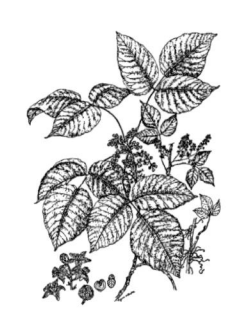

Leaflets three, let it be!

Poison ivy can look different in different situations. The key is that each leaf is made up of 3 distinct leaflets (*"Leaflets three, let it be!"*). Sometimes the leaf edges are notched, sometimes they're not. It can grow in almost any situation, full sun to full shade. If it has something to climb, like a tree trunk, it acts like a vine and can develop a wide, fuzzy, ropy stem. In full sun, it can grow almost like a shrub. In the fall, the leaves turn deep red-orange. Poison ivy can flower and may have white, waxy berries. Virginia creeper and boxelder tree are two plants that are sometimes mistaken for poison ivy.

Take the following precautions around poison ivy:

- Wear long sleeves, long pants, and gloves. Handle your clothes as little as possible afterwards, preferably wearing gloves. Keep "poison ivy-contaminated" clothes separate from other family laundry and wash them as soon as possible. Don't forget to wash or wipe down shoes too.
- As soon as possible after exposure:
  (1) Clean the exposed skin with rubbing alcohol.
  (2) Wash the area with cool water (do not use soap).
  (3) Shower with soap and warm water. (Using soap before step 3 can spread the poison ivy oils on your skin.)
- Consider a preventive lotion, especially if you're highly sensitive to poison ivy. One is IvyBlock®, a nonprescription lotion that is applied before any potential exposure to poison ivy. Its white, clay-like coating acts as a skin shield to prevent reactions in most susceptible people.
- Clean tools and equipment that have been exposed to poison ivy by rinsing them in cold water and wiping them down with alcohol or vinegar (be sure to wear rubber gloves). Tecnu® is a commercial outdoor skin cleaner that will remove plant oils from skin, clothing, and tools. People have been

known to get poison ivy up to a year later from oils remaining on clothes or tools.
- Don't try to burn poison ivy. The oils in the smoke can volatilize and still cause a reaction to skin or the lungs if inhaled.

Poison oak and poison sumac are poisonous plants similar to poison ivy, but less common. The same precautions are necessary if you are working around any of these plants.

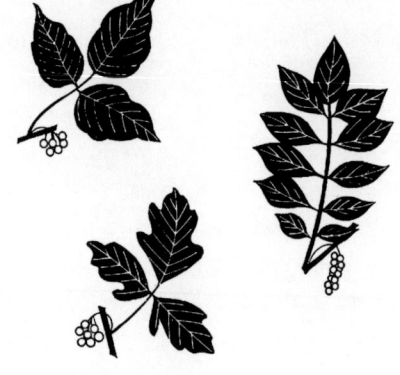

Poison ivy (upper left), poison sumac (upper right), and poison oak (bottom) all contain similar irritating oils

Key Points to Remember—Poison Ivy

- √ *"Leaflets three, let it be!" Poison ivy can look different in different situations, but each leaf is made up of 3 distinct leaflets.*
- √ *Wear long sleeves, long pants, and gloves when working around poison ivy.*
- √ *Keep "poison ivy-contaminated" clothes separate from other family laundry and wash them as soon as possible.*
- √ *As soon as possible after exposure, clean the exposed skin with rubbing alcohol, then wash the area with cool water (no soap), and finally shower with soap and warm water, in that order.*
- √ *People have been known to get poison ivy up to a year later from oils remaining on clothes or tools.*
- √ *Don't burn poison ivy.*

POWER-DUSTING AND POWER-SPRAYING

Powered pesticide application equipment can increase exposure hazard to applicators as compared to hand equipment. With power equipment, more pesticide is applied over a given time interval. Higher application pressures mean increased risk of leaks, splash-back, airborne residues, and drift, including drift back onto the applicator. Powered equipment is more complex and has more components that can fail without proper maintenance. A catastrophic equipment failure such as a burst fitting or a split hose can dose an applicator with a large volume of pesticide. Power equipment can apply spray or dust deep into hidden areas. There, unseen flames and pilot lights or spark-producing electrical equipment could ignite a flammable pesticide spray or dust and cause a fire or an explosion.

You can reduce your risk of pesticide exposure when using power sprayers and dusters through good maintenance of equipment and by following proper safety procedures.

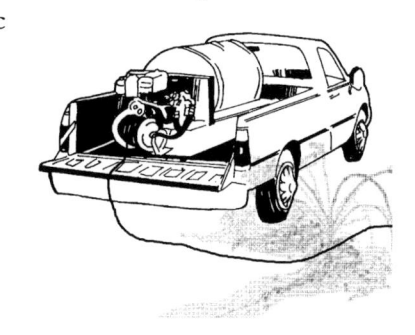

High application pressures increase the risk of catastrophic equipment failures

Equipment Inspection and Maintenance

Power equipment should be inspected before each use. Check for cracked, split, or damaged hoses (see discussion of replacing a damaged hose under *Spills*), cracked fittings, broken regulators and gauges, damaged tanks, and any other signs of defect or wear. Check oil and water levels in gasoline-powered engines. Power equipment inspection is also a good time to lubricate fittings and do other simple non-shop maintenance.

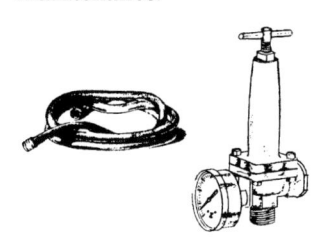

Hoses and fittings should be rated for maximum pump pressure

High pressure pumps usually need a pressure relief valve on the discharge side to prevent damage from high pressure buildup if the pump discharge happens to be blocked or closed. Set bypass and other valves properly and check that no lines are plugged or hoses kinked. Start up the unit and let it run for a few minutes, checking for leaks and making sure the equipment is operating properly before beginning your application.

Pest Control Technician Safety Manual

To help you keep power equipment in a safe operating condition, put together an inspection checklist for each power sprayer and power duster that you use.

All power equipment should get periodic shop maintenance as recommended by the manufacturer (oil, filter, lube changes, etc.). If any components need replacement, (and if you are authorized to do the work), use only hoses, pipes, and fittings that are rated for the maximum pump pressure. Before service, disconnect electric power, release all pressure, and drain all pesticide liquids from sprayers. In some cases, you may also need to remove pesticide dust from a duster before you service it.

A sample maintenance checklist for termite rigs is provided on the next page.

Precautions When Using Power Sprayers and Dusters

To reduce your exposure hazard when using power application equipment, wear personal protective equipment (PPE) such as a respirator, gloves, boots, eye protection, and a hat. Be careful around moving parts, such as shafts and pulleys, so that your clothing or body parts are not entangled. Do not remove guards. Do not operate a gasoline-driven sprayer in an enclosed or unventilated area.

For high-pressure pumps, secure the discharge line before starting; otherwise, it could whip around and cause injury or damage. Never use pressures higher than the maximum recommended by the manufacturer, or run pumps faster than the maximum recommended speed.

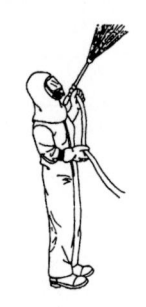

Wear plenty of PPE when power-spraying

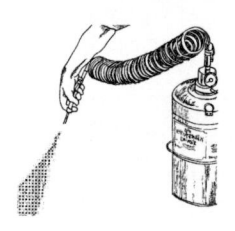

Apply dusts or sprays to the side or walk away from the application

For either dusts or sprays, apply the pesticide to the side (at a right angle to the direction you are walking) or walk backwards <u>away</u> from the direction of application so that you avoid splashback and do not walk through the pesticide you just applied. Keep application pressures as low as practical to avoid airborne residues, drift to nontarget areas, and splashback. For liquid applications, use a nozzle that produces large droplets to minimize air residues or wear a respirator and goggles. Be particularly careful in restricted spaces (sees *Attics and Crawlspaces*). Watch out for electrical circuits when spraying liquids, and pilot lights and other open flames when applying flammable materials.

| 146 |

Maintenance Checklist for Termite Rigs

Termite rigs must be maintained properly to operate safely and effectively. Follow the manufacturer's instructions for maintaining the pump, tank, engine and peripherals (flow meter, application tools, etc.), as well as the checklist below for daily, weekly, and seasonal maintenance. In the blank spaces, fill in any additional maintenance actions that are required by the manufacturer or your company.

Daily—

- ❏ Check oil
- ❏ Inspect starter rope
- ❏ Check engine for leaks
- ❏ Check pump lubrication
- ❏ Check hoses/clamps
- ❏ Inspect tank/plumbing
- ❏ Operational check
- ❏ Flush screens/lines/flow meter after use
- ❏ _____
- ❏ _____
- ❏ _____

Weekly—

- ❏ Check air filter
- ❏ Inspect carburetor throat and back plate for dirt
- ❏ Check muffler
- ❏ Unroll hose, unkink it, and check it for weak spots
- ❏ Clean tank
- ❏ Lubricate hose reel
- ❏ Check calibration
- ❏ _____
- ❏ _____
- ❏ _____

End of Season—

- ❏ Change oil
- ❏ Change spark plug
- ❏ Clean/change air filter
- ❏ Winterize engine (drain fuel, coat inside tank and cylinder with WD40, etc.)
- ❏ Do all manufacturer recommended pump maintenance
- ❏ Flush all lines and pump (for winter storage flush with 50/50 water & antifreeze)
- ❏ Check all bolts
- ❏ _____
- _____
- ❏ _____
- ❏ _____
- ❏ _____

Vehicle number _____ Responsible Technician _____

If a dust or liquid is flammable, put out all flames and pilot lights, and shut down all spark-producing equipment. Nonflammable materials can also cause a problem by extinguishing pilot lights.

Before opening the tank of a compressed-air power duster, be sure to release the air to prevent dust from blowing all over you. (For most units, releasing the air is accomplished by turning it upside down and opening the discharge valve.) When injecting dust into voids near electrical wiring, use a nonconducting tip to avoid electric shock.

Key Points to Remember—Power-Dusting & Spraying

- √ **Power dusting or spray equipment should be inspected before each use.**
- √ **Do not operate a gasoline-driven sprayer in an enclosed or unventilated area.**
- √ **Apply the pesticide to the side or walk backwards away from the direction of application.**
- √ **Higher application pressures mean increased risk of leaks, splashback, airborne residues, and drift, including drift back onto the applicator.**
- √ **Before opening the tank of a compressed-air power duster, be sure to release the air to prevent dust from blowing all over you.**

RADIATION

Radiation is used on an ever increasing scale in medicine, dentistry, and industry. Main users of man-made radiation include: medical facilities such as hospitals and pharmaceutical facilities; research and teaching institutions; nuclear reactors and their supporting facilities such as uranium mills and fuel preparation plants; and federal facilities involved in nuclear weapons production as part of their normal operation.

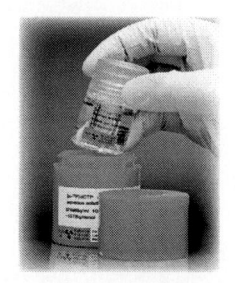

Radioactive materials are common in medical facilities

Photo © Andrei Tchernov/iStockphoto

Many of these facilities generate some radioactive waste; and some release a controlled amount of radiation into the environment. Radioactive materials are also used in common consumer products such as digital and luminous-dial wristwatches, ceramic glazes, and smoke detectors.

Health Effects of Radiation Exposure

Depending on the level of exposure and its duration, radiation can pose a health risk. It can adversely affect individuals directly exposed as well as their descendants. Radiation can affect cells of the body, increasing the risk of cancer or harmful genetic mutations that can be passed on to future generations; or, if the dosage is large enough to cause massive tissue damage, it may lead to death within a few weeks of exposure.

Minimizing Radiation Exposure

If you work in medical facilities, laboratories, or other sites that use radiation, be aware of potential risks. Do not work in radiation areas unless you have been authorized to do so, and unless you have been trained in the appropriate protective measures to minimize the risks.

There are three basic ways to reduce exposure to radiation.

- Avoid being close to radiation sources.
- Reduce the time spent near a source of radiation.
- Place shielded barriers between you and the radiation source.

Signs and Posting

Areas or materials with radiation hazards are typically identified by one or more of the following:

- Signs that have the standard radiation symbol (trefoil) colored magenta or black on a yellow background.
- Yellow and magenta rope, tape, chains or other barriers to designate the boundaries of posted areas.
- Tags and labels with a yellow background and either a magenta or black standard radiation symbol to identify radioactive material.
- Yellow plastic wrapping or a labeled container around a package containing radioactive material.
- Designated radiation storage areas.

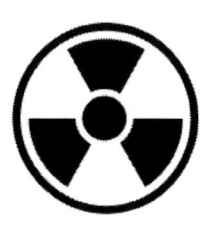

Radiation symbol

Graphic © Dale Taylor/ iStockphoto

Pest Control Technician Safety Manual

Sites with radiation hazards are often posted to designate the level of risk. Typical sign wording might be "radiation control area" or "radiation buffer area" or "radiation area" or "radioactive materials area" or "airborne radioactive materials area."

A "controlled area" may surround an area with actual radiation hazards. Typically, there are no significant radiation hazards in the controlled area itself. Do not enter controlled areas unless you are authorized to do so.

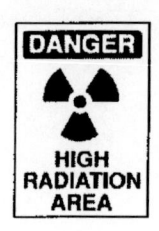

A "radiation buffer area" may be established within the controlled area to provide a secondary boundary for minimizing exposures. Typically, you will not be allowed to enter a buffer area unless you are continuously escorted or have received special safety training.

The highest risk areas will be designated as "radiation areas," "radioactive material areas," "airborne radioactive materials areas," or similar. Never enter these areas without special authorization and training. Even then, you may need to be escorted.

Highest risk areas will be designated "radiation areas"

Monitoring

Since radiation cannot be detected with any of the human senses, special detection devices may be required when working in or near radiation areas. Most commonly, film badges are used to monitor occupational exposure to radiation. They are worn between the waist and head on the front of the body, with the label side of the film badge facing the source of radiation. The badges are periodically turned in so that your level of radiation exposure, if any, can be measured.

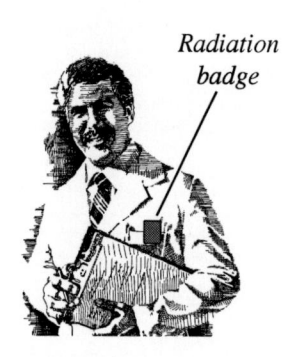

Film badges measure radiation exposure

Precautions When Working Around Radiation

- Obey all signs/postings.
- Comply with all radiation safety rules.
- Be careful around radiation waste collection containers in medical labs, hospitals, and other medical facilities.
- Do not enter radiation areas unless authorized to do so and properly trained.

- If working in a radiation area with an escort, always obey the instructions of your escort.
- Wear a radiation badge if required to do so.
- When in doubt about radiation safety, report to an authorized individual for instruction.

Key Points to Remember—Radiation

- √ **Radiation may pose a health risk to you and to your descendants.**
- √ **The standard radiation symbol is a trefoil colored magenta or black on a yellow background.**
- √ **Never enter radiation areas without authorization and training.**
- √ **When in doubt about radiation safety, report to an authorized individual for instruction.**

RODENTS

You have a number of personal health and safety concerns when controlling rodents: bites and scratches, ectoparasites (fleas, ticks, mites, lice), allergies, and disease. These concerns obviously overlap, because, for example, you can catch a rodent-borne disease from being bitten by a rodent (ratbite fever) or from a rodent's ticks or fleas (Lyme disease or plague). The safety precautions you take will depend on the species of rodent and on where you work. If you work in a hantavirus area or a Lyme disease area you will need to take special precautions against these diseases. Make sure you know the incidence of these diseases in your region and what safety precautions are necessary. If you don't, ask your supervisor.

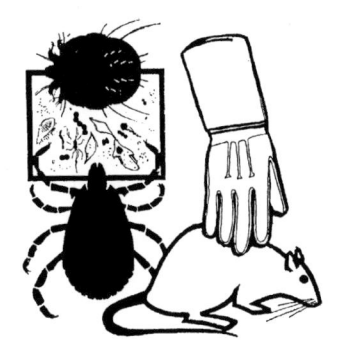

Potential health risks from rodents include bites, allergy, ectoparasites, and disease

Rodent Bites and Scratches

Rodents, and in particular rats, have long incisor teeth and can give you a nasty bite. They are aggressive when cornered or handled, and will try to bite and scratch. If you need to handle live rodents, wear animal-handling gloves or trappers' gloves. Live rats are normally lifted by grasping the whole body--palm over back and side with forefinger behind the head and the thumb and second finger extending the forelimbs so that they may be controlled. Use your other hand to grasp the tail to keep the rat stretched out. Mice are usually caught and lifted by the tail, about two-thirds of the way up from the base.

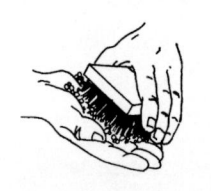

Wash the wound with soap and water and let it bleed

If you are bitten or scratched by a rodent, immediately wash the wound with soap and water. Clean the bite by allowing it to bleed. Be sure to see a physician. Wild rodents can transmit diseases such as ratbite fever, and cause other infections, including tetanus. Rabies, however, is not considered a hazard of rodent bites.

Ectoparasites

Rodents harbor a wide range of ectoparasites including fleas, ticks, mites, and lice. Some can transmit disease to pets, wildlife, and people (Lyme disease, typhus, and plague). Some rodent ectoparasites will move onto people. The tropical rat mite is the most common ectoparasite of roof rats in some areas, including southern California. Its bite causes irritation and sometimes a painful skin condition. The mouse mite leaves its host, a house mouse, after feeding and climbs onto walls, where it may then move onto pets or people.

Be alert to the risk of ectoparasites when controlling heavy populations of rodents. You, too, can be attacked. Use repellents when necessary and wear gloves. In heavy infestations, consider treating the area with an insecticide/acaricide before beginning your control program.

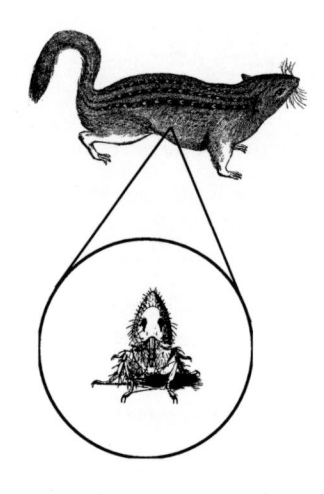

Fleas and other ectoparasites can move from rodents and bite you

Pest Control Technician Safety Manual

Rodent Allergy

See the discussion of *Mouse Allergy* in the *Allergy* section.

Rodent-borne Diseases

See also *Tick-transmitted Diseases* for Lyme disease.

Hantavirus

Hantavirus is a rare but often fatal disease caused by a virus most commonly carried by the deer mouse (*Peromyscus maniculatus*) and, in some areas, other species of mice such as the whitefooted mouse (*P. leucopus*). Through August 24, 2006, a total of 451 cases of hantavirus pulmonary syndrome (HPS) have been reported in the United States. Thirty-six percent of all reported cases have resulted in death. About three-quarters of patients with HPS have been residents of rural areas.

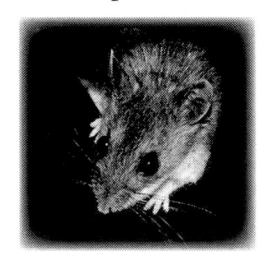

Deer mice and whitefooted mice are hantavirus hosts

Photo © K. Garrenson/iStockphoto

While rare, hantavirus is of special concern because of its high fatality rate. The disease begins with flu-like symptoms, but the lungs begin to fill with fluid, and death from respiratory failure can be rapid. The virus has been documented in 30 states, with the majority of cases in the western United States. The virus is spread through the urine, saliva, or feces of rodents (particularly the deer mouse but also the white-footed mouse in some areas of the country), most often when the virus becomes airborne and then is inhaled.

If you are regularly exposed to rodents in suspected hantavirus areas you should follow the special recommendations of the Centers for Disease Control (CDC). As of this writing, those recommendations include medical monitoring, using a respirator with a "HE" (High Efficiency) filter (any N100, R100, or P100 filter is classified as an HE filter) and gloves when removing rodents from traps or handling rodents, washing and disinfecting gloves before removing them, and regularly disinfecting traps and other rodent equipment.

Traps, gloves, and other items can be disinfected with a general household disinfectant followed by soap and water. A hypochlorite solution prepared by mixing three tablespoons of household bleach in one gallon of water may be used in place of a commercial disinfectant.

Disinfect traps, gloves, and other equipment

| 153 |

In hantavirus areas you should dispose of rodent carcasses by placing them in a plastic bag containing a sufficient amount of a general-purpose household disinfectant to thoroughly wet the carcasses. Seal the bag and then dispose of it by burying in a two-foot deep hole or by burning. If burying or burning are not feasible, contact your local or state health department about other appropriate disposal methods.

These recommendations generally apply in areas that have had problems with hantavirus. Be aware, however, that hantavirus may appear anywhere, and take precautions when working in accounts that are or may have been infested with deer mice. Be particularly careful in attics, crawls, and outbuildings in rural and suburban areas. Always wear a respirator and use gloves if you believe there is risk of hantavirus. Note that the virus can be present in dust and debris even after infestations of deer mice have been eliminated.

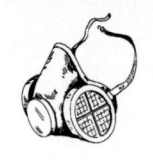

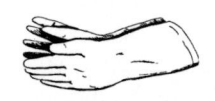

Wear respirator and gloves where there is risk of hantavirus

Typical mouse control programs aimed at the house mouse probably do not require the use of respirators, but you should still wear gloves and take care when servicing traps and bait stations. Wear a respirator with an HE filter whenever cleaning up or otherwise disturbing large accumulations of rodent droppings.

LCM — Lymphocytic Choriomeningitis

It's a mouthful. *Lymphocytic choriomeningitis*, or LCM, is a virus that is spread to people primarily by the common house mouse, *Mus musculus*. Infection rates in mice range from 3 to 40%. Other rodents such as guinea pigs, gerbils, or hamsters can become infected if they are exposed to the virus in pet stores or homes.

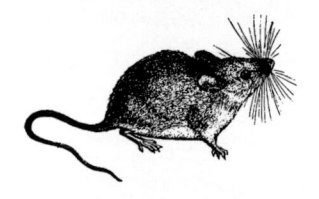

LCM is a virus spread to people by the house mouse

LCM made news recently when four organ transplant recipients were found to have been infected with the virus from a single organ donor. An investigation traced the source of the virus to a pet hamster purchased by the donor from a pet store. Three percent of the animals tested in the store were found to carry LCM.

People become infected with LCM when rodent urine, droppings, saliva or nest material come into contact with broken skin, the nose, eyes, or mouth, or if they are bitten by an infected rodent.

In people with normal immune systems, LCM often shows few or no symptoms. People that do become ill generally have flu-like symptoms at first. The disease can progress with symptoms of meningitis (fever, headache, stiff neck) or encephalitis (inflammation of the brain). Most people recover completely. Some studies have indicated that approximately 5% of people in urban areas are infected with LCM. There apparently is no person-to-person transmission of the disease other than from mother to fetus or through organ transplants.

Lymphocytic choriomeningitis is currently considered to be a rare disease.

LCM Safety Precautions

The precautions for LCM are basically the same as those you would take to protect yourself from hantavirus. The Centers for Disease Control advises the following:

- Wear rubber, latex, vinyl, or nitrile gloves when doing rodent control. After removing gloves, wash hands with soap and water.
- Avoid stirring up dust or mouse droppings. If cleaning up a mouse-infested site, wet down droppings and the contaminated area with a disinfectant solution.
- Spray dead rodents with disinfect and double-bag rodents, nest material, and cleaning materials for disposal.
- People who have pet hamsters, guinea pigs, or other rodents should be sure to wash their hands after handling the pet or after cleaning cages.

Plague

Before modern medicine and pest control, outbreaks of plague, also called the "Black Death," periodically killed millions of people. Today, plague is rare and can be treated with antibiotics, although it remains a potentially deadly disease. In 2006, there were 13 confirmed cases of human plague in the U.S. among residents of four states: New Mexico (7), Colorado (3), California (2), and Texas (1). This was the largest number of plague cases since 1994. Two of the cases were fatal.

Plague is spread by the bite of an infected flea or by handling an infected animal. While plague was once primarily an urban disease attributed to city rats, almost all cases today occur in Arizona, California, Colorado, New Mexico, and Texas. These cases are traced to prairie dogs, ground squirrels, other

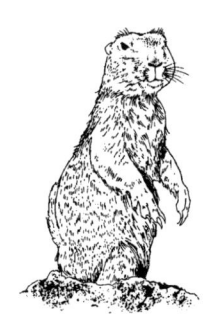

Prairie dogs, other wild rodents, rabbits and hares may carry plague in the western U.S.

wild rodents, rabbits or hares, as well as animals, such as pet dogs, that have come in contact with wildlife and then become infested with their infected fleas.

In plague areas, the Centers for Disease Control advises removing rodent food and harborage, and avoiding sick or dead animals. Pest control technicians, trappers, and wildlife researchers should use insect repellents, wear protective clothing and gloves when handling trapped animals, and stay away from wild animal nests where fleas may be waiting for a new host.

Ratbite Fever

Ratbite fever (RBF) is a rare, systemic bacterial illness that can be caused by a bite or scratch from a rodent, or by ingesting food or water contaminated with rat feces. Cases have also been recorded as a result of bites from mice, squirrels, and gerbils, and from contact with dogs or cats that fed on these animals.

Ratbite fever begins with flu-like symptoms and an irregular, relapsing fever. Within a couple of days, a rash develops on the palms and soles of the feet. Patients are treated with antibiotics and most cases clear up within two weeks, but 13% of untreated cases are fatal, which is certainly another good reason to wear gloves when handling rodents.

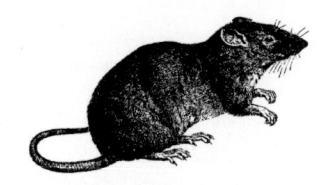

Rats, mice, and other rodents can transmit ratbite fever

Guidelines for Handling Rodents

- If handling live rodents, wear animal-handling gloves or trapper's gloves.
- Wear gloves when handling dead rodents.
- Dispose of rodent carcasses by placing them in a sealed plastic bag. If you are working in an area with suspected rodent-borne disease, add a sufficient amount of a general-purpose household disinfectant to thoroughly wet the carcasses (a hypochlorite solution prepared by mixing three tablespoons of household bleach in one gallon of water may be used in place of a commercial disinfectant).
- If working in an area of heavy rodent infestation, consider spraying the area with an insecticide/acaracide to eliminate ectoparasites.
- In Lyme disease or plague areas, spray yourself with DEET or other insect/tick repellent.

Guidelines for Cleaning Up Rodent-Infested Sites

Hantavirus, LCM, and various allergies are associated with the saliva, urine, and feces of rodents. Many technicians provide services to clean up rodent-infested sites. If you provide clean-up services, protect yourself with PPE, and try and prevent rodent-contaminated dirt or dust from becoming airborne. Here are some specific guidelines to follow:

- Wear rubber, latex, vinyl, or nitrile gloves. Wear a respirator with an HE filter (N-100, R-100, or P-100).
- Use a paper towel to pick up rodent droppings and urine. Place the paper towel in the garbage.
- Before you handle them, spray dead rodents and rodent nests with a disinfectant or a chlorine (1:10) solution, soaking them thoroughly.
- Place the dead rodent or rodent nest in a plastic bag, seal the bag, then place it into a second plastic bag and seal that bag. Dispose of the double bags by discarding them in a covered trash can that is regularly emptied, or by burning or burying the bags.
- Disinfect any items or areas that might have been contaminated by the rodents or their urine or droppings. Do not vacuum or sweep rodent urine, droppings, or contaminated surfaces until they have been disinfected.
- Wearing gloves, use a disinfectant or chlorine solution to mop floors, disinfect countertops, cabinets, drawers, and other surfaces. Use a disinfectant or commercial-grade steam cleaner or shampooer to clean carpets and upholstered furniture. Any bedding or clothing that may have been contaminated should be laundered in hot water and detergent.
- Items that can't be easily cleaned should be left outdoors in sunlight for several hours or in an area free of rodents for at least one week. After that time, the virus should no longer be infectious.
- Disinfect gloves before removing them. Use a disinfectant or soap and water. After you remove your gloves, wash your hands with soap and water.

Disinfect areas contaminated by rodents or their urine or droppings

Key Points to Remember—Rodents

- √ You have 4 primary health concerns when controlling rodents: (1) bites and scratches, (2) ectoparasites, (3) allergy, and (4) disease.
- √ Wear gloves when handling rodents; if the rodents are alive, wear animal-handling gloves or trappers' gloves.
- √ Dispose of rodent carcasses by placing them in a plastic bag.
- √ Hantavirus is spread through the urine, saliva, or feces of rodents (particularly the deer mouse), most often when the virus is inhaled.
- √ Hantavirus can be present in dust and debris even after infestations of deer mice have been eliminated.
- √ Always wear a respirator with an HE filter whenever cleaning up or otherwise disturbing large accumulations of rodent droppings.
- √ LCM (lymphocytic choriomeningitis) is a viral disease that is spread to people primarily by the house mouse.
- √ Ratbite fever (RBF) is a rare disease usually caused by a bite or scratch of a rodent.
- √ Plague is spread by the bite of an infected flea or by handling an infected animal.
- √ Prevent rodent-contaminated dirt or dust from becoming airborne during clean-up.

ROOFS

If you birdproof or batproof buildings, if you remove nuisance animals from attics or chimneys, if you tarp buildings for fumigation, if you control wasps or bees or remove nests...you may find yourself up high on a roof, overhang, or ledge where a fall is a very real possibility. The Occupational Safety and Health Administration (OSHA) requires that workers on a roof, ledge, beam, cornice, or similar site where there is a risk of injury from falling, be protected by a fall protection system.

Do not work on roofs or other sites where there is a risk of falling more than six feet unless you have been trained to recognize fall hazards and how to minimize them, and how to safely use a body harness fall protection system. If there are no guardrails, safety lines, or other fall protection systems in place on a roof, ledge, or similar worksite, you will need to wear a body harness fall protection system. The system includes a body harness, lanyard, rope grab, safety line, anchor, and various rings and connector clips.

Be sure to inspect all components of the body harness system for mildew, wear, damage, and other deterioration before EACH use. Any deteriorated or damaged components need to be withdrawn from service immediately.

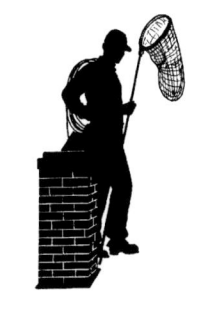

If you work on roofs or ledges, you must be protected from falls

How to Put on a Safety Harness in 10 Easy Steps

Refer to the instructions that came with your harness, since your harness may have some special characteristics. In most cases, you should proceed as follows:

1. Inspect your harness carefully.
2. Hold the harness by the D-ring at the back.
3. Shake the harness so the straps fall into place.
4. Open all buckles.
5. Slip the straps over your shoulders. Make sure the D-ring is located between your shoulder blades.
6. Pull each leg strap up between your legs and connect.
7. Connect the waist strap (if so equipped).
8. Connect the chest strap so that it is at mid-chest and tighten so that the shoulder straps are snug and secure.
9. Tighten all buckles for a snug fit.
10. Pass excess straps through loop keepers.

Rig your fall protection system so that you cannot free-fall more than six feet, nor contact any lower level or objects, and to avoid swing fall injuries (injury caused by a pendulum swing at the end of a fall). Check that the anchor point is safe (able to support at least 5,000 pounds), the safety line is adequate, the rope grab is installed in the proper direction to lock in the event of a fall, the lanyard is properly

Pest Control Technician Safety Manual

connected, the harness correctly adjusted, and all clips and connectors are closed shut.

If the work site is more than 25 feet above the ground and if the use of safety harnesses and lanyards or more conventional types of protection are not practical, an approved safety net must be installed instead.

Under certain conditions, you do not need a fall protection system even though you are at risk of injury from falling:

(1) if you are working on a ladder, or
(2) if the work is of short duration and limited exposure, or
(3) if installing the fall protection system is just as hazardous as doing the job itself.

Numbers two and three appear to apply to some pest control work such as going up on a roof to inspect for pests or to place traps. Ask your supervisor for guidance. In all cases, however, you still must be aware of the dangers, work safely, and be under adequate supervision. If you work in high places, be sure you are trained in how to protect yourself from falls.

You also need to avoid electric shock from roof-level power lines, which may be unprotected or damaged, and rooftop electrical equipment. See *Electric Shock* and *Ladders*.

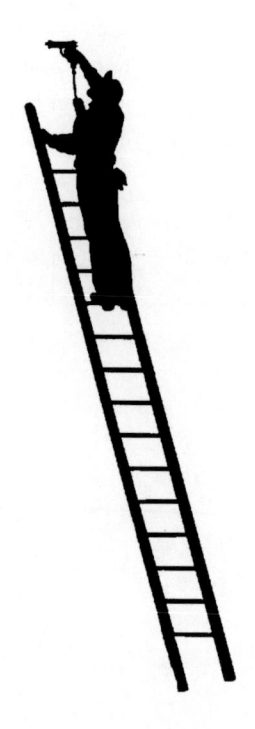

You do not need a fall protection system while working on a ladder

Key Points to Remember—Roofs

- √ **Do not work on roofs or other sites where there is a risk of falling more than six feet unless you have been trained to recognize fall hazards and how to minimize them.**
- √ **A fall protection system is a device or system that will keep you from falling more than six feet before being caught.**
- √ **Fall protection systems include roofing slide guards, guardrails, body harness systems, and nets.**
- √ **Inspect all components of a body harness system before each use.**

√ **You will not need a fall protection system if: (1) you are working on a ladder, or (2) the work is of short duration and limited exposure, or (3) installing the fall protection system is just as hazardous as doing the job itself.**

√ **Avoid roof-level power lines and rooftop electrical equipment.**

SCAFFOLDS

Each year, more than 60 workers are killed by falls from scaffolds. Some pest control technicians work on scaffolds, particularly for bird work. The scaffolds are either supported (usually by posts/beams and legs) or suspended (by ropes).

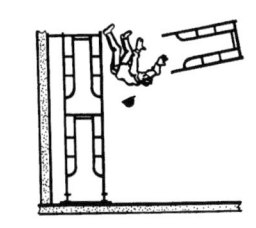

Do not work on a scaffold unless you have had scaffold safety training

To work safely on a scaffold you must be able to recognize possible hazards and understand safety procedures. Do not work on a scaffold unless you have been trained in the proper use of a scaffold, how to get on and off of it, electrical hazards, fall protection, protection against falling objects, determining maximum safe load, proper handling of materials on the scaffold, proper scaffold construction, and site safety.

Never work on a scaffold during storms or high winds or when it is covered with ice or snow. Make sure you do not allow tools, materials, and junk to accumulate on a scaffold. If a scaffold is more than 10 feet above a level, you need to have some kind of fall protection, such as a safety harness (see discussion in *Roofs*). A "competent person" must inspect a scaffold before each workshift and after anything happens that could affect the scaffold, structure, ground, or flooring.

Scaffold Standards

All scaffolds and their supports need to be capable of supporting their load with a fourfold safety factor. All planking must be "scaffold-grade," as recognized by grading rules for the type of wood used. Maximum permissible spans for scaffold planks are shown in the table on the next page.

The maximum permissible span for $1^1/_4$ x 9-inch or wider plank for full thickness is four feet, with medium loading of 50 pounds per square foot. Scaffold planks need to extend over their end supports not less than six inches or more than 18 inches. Scaffold planking must be overlapped a minimum of 12 inches or secured from movement. Wood planks must be unpainted, so any cracks can be easily seen.

Planking Specifications for Scaffolds

	Full Thickness[1] Undressed Lumber			Nominal Thickness[2] Lumber	
Working load (p.s.f.)	25	50	75	25	50
Permissible span (ft.)	10	8	6	8	6

1/ Undressed lumber measures its full size: a 2x10-inch board measures 2 inches by 10 inches.

2/ Finished lumber does not measure its labeled size: after it has been planed and finished, a board sold as a 2x10 actually measures $1^1/_2$ inches x $9^1/_4$ inches.

Railings and toe boards need to be installed on all open sides and ends of platforms that are more than ten feet above the ground. However, they are not required when the scaffold is entirely within the interior of a building if the scaffold (1) covers the entire floor area of any room, and (2) does not have any side exposed to a hoistway, elevator shaft, stairwell, or other floor openings.

There also must be a screen with $1/_2$-inch maximum openings between the toe-board and the guardrail where persons are required to work or pass under the scaffold. If a scaffold is more than 2 feet above or below a level, there must be a way to get on or off — such as a ladder, ramp, or personnel hoist. It must not be more than 14" horizontally from the scaffold. Keep scaffolds ten feet or more from power lines (or three feet, if lines are less than 300 volts), unless you are sure the power lines are de-energized.

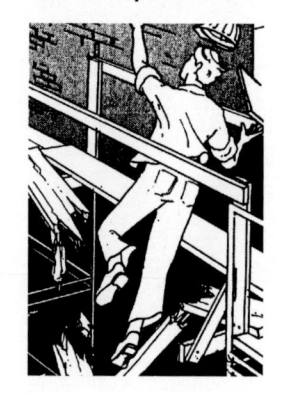

Substandard planking is a major cause of falls and injuries from scaffolds

Key Points to Remember—Scaffolds

- √ **All scaffolds and their supports need to be capable of supporting their load with a fourfold safety factor.**
- √ **All planking must be scaffold-grade.**
- √ **Scaffold planks need to extend over their end supports not less than six inches nor more than 18 inches.**
- √ **Scaffold planking must be overlapped a minimum of 12 inches or secured from movement.**
- √ **If a scaffold is more than 10 feet above a level, you need to have some kind of fall protection.**
- √ **Do not work on a scaffold (1) if you haven't been trained, (2) during storms or high winds, or (3) when the scaffold is covered with ice or snow.**

SLIPS, TRIPS, AND FALLS

About 10 percent of all accidents causing lost time from work are due to slips, trips, or falls. OSHA requires that employers <u>and</u> employees take certain precautions to prevent such accidents.

The possibility of an injury from a fall is not limited to your company's facilities. You're more likely to trip or slip in an unfamiliar location such as a customer's home, a food warehouse, even walking from your truck to the front door of an account.

Much of slip and fall prevention is basic and obvious, but it doesn't hurt to review it now and then. Indoors, falls often occur in poorly lit areas like basements. Construction debris and stored items increase your chances of tripping. Condensation on surfaces can create a hazard in warm, damp areas like commercial kitchens, laundries, or boiler rooms. In garages, shops, and store rooms, spilled oil, grease, even spilled pesticide, can result in a slip. Even a little spilled water when you fill your spray tank can trip you up. Outdoors, falls are often weather-related. Snow, ice, even

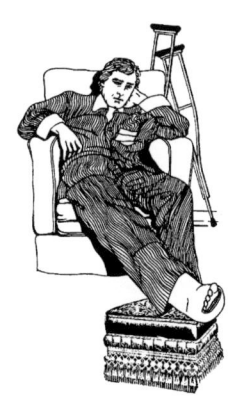

10% of all accidents causing lost time from work are due to slips, trips, or falls

rain, can make some surfaces treacherous, particularly if the surface is oily to begin with.

In the workplace, friction coatings on stairs, fluorescent paints, good lighting, and warning signs can help prevent falls. There are steps that you can take as well to make sure you don't become an injury statistic (see box below).

> ### How to Avoid Slips, Trips, and Falls
> - Carry a good, working flashlight when working in low light areas.
> - Wear skid-resistant shoes or boots.
> - Move slowly and carefully in unfamiliar places.
> - Pick up tools and equipment that are not in use.
> - Keep electrical cords and hoses away from walkways.
> - When carrying equipment, balance the load, and watch where you step.
> - Don't carry loads that block your vision.
> - Keep your hands on stair rails and ladders.
> - Walk, don't run, and watch where you're going.
> - Stay away from the edges of loading docks, manholes, roofs, and other edges.
> - Don't rush up or down stairs.
> - Be extra careful on stairs that are unusually steep or irregularly spaced.
> - Keep all four chair legs on the floor; don't rock backwards.
> - Don't leave drawers open.
> - Be careful of ice.
> - Clean up spills immediately.

Minimizing Injury During a Fall

How you fall and hit the ground determine the extent of your injury. If you find yourself falling, throw away anything in your hands. Forget the value of a tool, or whatever, and protect yourself. Toss it away so that you don't fall on it and it doesn't fall on you. Turn and roll. Don't land on your back or head, try to land rolling onto the large muscles of your thigh, buttocks, or upper back.

As you hit the ground, try to slap the ground and shout. Slapping the ground with your palm and inner forearm spreads impact. Shouting like a martial arts expert reduces internal compression from holding your breath. Relax after hitting the ground. You are more likely to roll and not crack your head or an elbow or knee.

Falls and Aging

As you age, you are more likely to slip, trip, or fall. Problems with balance, poor vision, dizziness, medications, and even syncope (drop attacks) all contribute to the increased injury rate in older workers. Furthermore, if you are an older worker injured in a fall, you will lose, on average, nearly twice as much time from work than would a younger worker. You are also more than twice as likely to sustain a fracture. If you are an older technician, you need to be especially careful to protect yourself from falling.

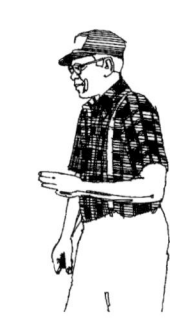

Older workers are more likely to fall and get injured

Key Points to Remember—Slips, Trips, and Falls

- √ **Carry a good, working flashlight when working in low light areas.**
- √ **Wear skid-resistant shoes or boots.**
- √ **Clean up spills immediately.**
- √ **If falling, toss away anything you are carrying, and turn and roll to minimize impact.**
- √ **As you age, you are more likely to slip, trip, or fall, and you are more than twice as likely to break a bone.**

SPILLS

A spill is any accidental release of pesticide. The spill may be minor, requiring little cleanup effort, or it may be major, involving large amounts of pesticide and serious contamination. You must know beforehand how to respond if you have a spill. Even a spill that appears minor can endanger you, other people, and the environment, especially if mishandled. Large leaks or spills require specially trained and equipped emergency crews. The early steps you take to control a spill can reduce or eliminate damage or injury. The faster you act, the less chance the spill will cause harm.

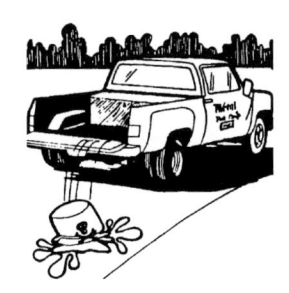

Large spills require specially trained emergency crews

Spill Management

Most pesticide spills are minor, just a dribble that can be easily cleaned up. But not always. In a spill emergency, remember the three C's...**C**ontrol, **C**ontain, **C**lean up. The order of the following steps may change depending on the toxicity of the pesticide, the size of the spill, and whether people are injured or contaminated.

The First "C"...Control

1. **Protect Yourself**—If the pesticide has spilled or sprayed on you, strip down, and wash down. Before you get near a pesticide spill, put on the appropriate personal protective equipment required by the label. If in doubt as to what's required, wear all of the protective equipment that you can: rubber gloves, goggles, respirator, boots, etc. If there are injuries, call for medical assistance. Move any injured people to a safe location away from the spill. Administer first aid. Wash down or decontaminate anyone who has come in contact with the pesticide.

2. **Stop the Source of the Spill**—If a pesticide container is leaking, place it inside a plastic bag or plastic bucket, ideally with a lid (see *Damaged Pesticide Container* following). If a hose bursts or is leaking, clamp or kink it, turn off the pump and release the pressure. If a spray tank is overflowing, stop the inflow and try to cap off the tank.

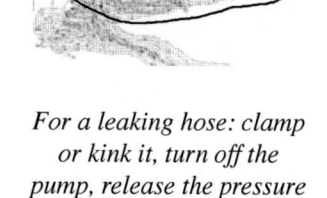

   For a leaking hose: clamp or kink it, turn off the pump, release the pressure

3. **Protect Others**—Keep onlookers at least 30 feet away from the spill site. If necessary, rope off the site or place barriers and warning signs. Keep people away from any fumes or drift. If you think the spill contains a highly volatile or explosive chemical, keep people even further back. In this case, don't allow anyone to smoke and don't light road flares.

4. **Stay at the Site**—Someone must remain at the spill site at all times until it is cleaned up. Don't leave the site unless you are replaced by a knowledgeable person wearing the proper protective equipment.

The Second "C"...Contain

1. **Contain the Spill**—As soon as you have stopped the source of the spill, take steps to contain it in as small an area as possible. Do whatever you can to keep the pesticide from spreading or running downhill. A very small

spill on level ground can be contained simply by applying a spill absorbent around it and directly onto it. For larger spills, use containment "snakes" to encircle the spill and hold it in place. Outdoors, you can also use a shovel to make either a trench or a dike of dirt around the spill to keep it from spreading. If you have no other alternatives, circle the spill with rags or paper towels.

2. **Protect Water Sources**—Act quickly if the spill could move towards a body of water such as a pond or stream, or if it is flowing in a direction where it could enter a ditch, storm drain, floor drain, well, or sinkhole. Immediately block or redirect any spill that is moving towards such an area.

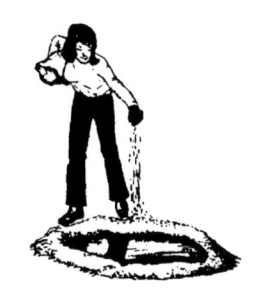

Keep the spill from spreading and flowing downhill

3. **Absorb Liquids, or Cover Dry Materials**— Once you have stopped the movement of the spill, absorb it or cover it. Liquid pesticide spills can be absorbed with various commercial products such as absorbent powders, spill pillows, or absorbent pads. You can also cover the spill with fine sand, sweeping compound, sawdust, clay, kitty litter, vermiculite, paper towels, or shredded newspapers. Work the absorbent into the spill by using a broom or shovel. Under windy conditions, a spill of a dry pesticide such as a dust, wettable powder, or granules can blow into nearby areas. In rainy weather, a dry spill can be activated or can turn into a liquid spill. If you can't sweep up a dry spill immediately, keep it from becoming airborne or rain-soaked by covering it with a sheet of plastic (use weights to hold down the plastic). Lightly misting a dry pesticide spill with water will also keep it from blowing, but if you use too much water, you may start pesticidal action or the spill may clump. If a dry pesticide clumps, it may come unusable, and it then will have to be disposed of as a hazardous material.

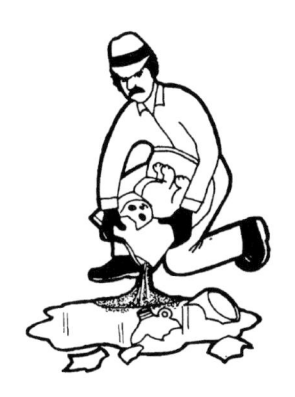

Use absorbent powders, pillows, pads, or kitty litter to absorb spills

The Third "C"...Clean Up

Once you have **controlled** and **contained** a pesticide spill, the final step is to **clean up** the spilled material and decontaminate the area and equipment.

1. **Pick Up Spilled Pesticide—** For spills of liquid pesticides, sweep up the pesticide and absorbent material and place it into a plastic bucket or heavy-duty plastic bag. Some commercial absorbents allow you to add the material, with water, to your spray tank and reuse it. Keep adding absorbent until all of the liquid is soaked up and swept up. For dry spills such as dusts, granules, or wettable powders, sweep up and reuse the pesticide if it is clean and dry. Wet or dirty material must be placed in a bucket or bag for disposal.

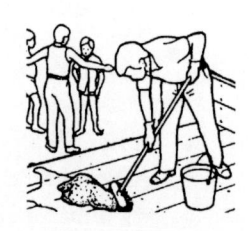

    Keep adding absorbent until all the liquid has been soaked up and swept up for disposal

2. **Decontaminate the Spill Site—** For large spills, contact the manufacturer for instructions. If the surface on which the pesticide has spilled is nonporous, such as sealed concrete, vinyl flooring, or ceramic tile, use water (or other diluent listed on the label) and a strong detergent to wash the area. Don't allow the wash water to run off of the site. Use absorbents again to soak up the wash water and place the collected material in a bucket or plastic bag. If the spill surface is porous like soil, unsealed wood, or carpet, you may have to remove the contaminated surface and dispose of it as you would excess pesticide. Some pesticide labels require that you also "neutralize" the spill site. Neutralizing may require repeat applications of bleach and hydrated lime, or the use of activated charcoal. Follow the manufacturer's instructions for neutralizing a spill.

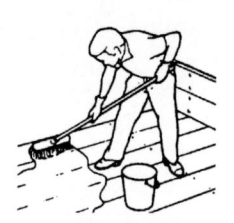

    Follow the manufacturer instructions for decontaminating the spill site

3. **Decontaminate Equipment—**Unless advised otherwise by the pesticide manufacturer, use a strong mixture of chlorine bleach, dishwasher detergent, and water to clean any vehicles or equipment that were contaminated by the spill or were used in the cleanup process. Clean personal protective equipment such as respirators and gloves according to manufacturer's instructions. Discard porous items such as clothing, brooms, and shoes that have become saturated with pesticide.

4. **Decontaminate Yourself** — When you have finished all other cleanup, wash yourself thoroughly with soap and water. Pay special attention to any exposed skin and always wash your face, neck, hands, and forearms.

Spill Assistance

When to call for assistance depends on whether you or others are injured or at immediate risk of injury or poisoning. Concern for your welfare and the public's should be your first priority. If there is no risk of injury, first control and contain the spill, then call for assistance. Even if you feel that no assistance is needed, many local and state authorities *require* that you notify police, fire department, or transportation department, etc. of a pesticide spill over a certain size. The same is true for many federal sites, universities, cities, and other municipalities. Be sure that you know what spill reporting is required in your work area <u>before</u> you have a spill.

As soon as the spill is under control, call your office or supervisor and explain the situation. The office may give you instructions and make the necessary contact calls for you, or direct you to call authorities yourself. If company policy is for you to contact the authorities, then have a list of contact phone numbers in your vehicle.

Who to Call in Case of a Spill

- **If you or anyone else may have been poisoned by exposure to the pesticide** - Call 911 for emergency assistance and provide rescue workers or the hospital emergency room with label information regarding brand name, active ingredient, manufacturer's phone number, signs and symptoms of poisoning and antidotes.
- **If the spill may expose the public to pesticide residues** - Call the proper regulatory agency or the local health department.
- **If the spill occurs on a highway** - Call the highway patrol, state police, or the highway department.
- **If you suspect that the spill is flammable** - Call the fire department with information under *"Physical or Chemical Hazards"* on the label.
- **If the spill occurs on a county road or city street** - Call the county sheriff, city police, or fire department.

Some pest control companies have arrangements with the Chemical Transportation Emergency Center - **CHEMTREC** at **1-800-262-8200** (hotline available 24-hours a day for *spill emergencies only*) or **INFOTRAC** at **1-800-535-5053**. Your state may have its own spill reporting hotline that you must call within a certain time period (two hours from the time of the spill, for example). Whoever you call, have the product label at hand.

Most pesticide labels or MSDSs will list an emergency phone number that will put you in direct contact with the manufacturer or other organizations or people who know how to manage emergencies for that product.

Once the spill is under control, or has been cleaned up, fill out an incident report of the spill. Provide a description in chronological order of what happened, where it happened, who was involved, and the actions you took. Be factual; avoid placing blame or making assumptions (see *Accident Reporting*).

Spill Control Kit

A pest control service vehicle should carry a special spill control kit to clean up a pesticide spill. Even if you do only in-house pest control and don't use a vehicle, you still need a spill control kit. There are commercial kits available from pest control suppliers. You can also put together your own. Here's what a spill control kit should contain:

1. A plastic jug of clean water to wash pesticide off of skin or to rinse eyes. You can't count on having a garden hose or a shower nearby.
2. A small bottle of detergent for washing pesticide from skin and for washing the spill area after cleanup.
3. Coveralls or a clean change of clothes. Never continue to wear clothes on which you've spilled pesticide.
4. Fifty feet of twine and stakes to rope off a large spill area, and warning signs or warning flags.
5. Rubber gloves and rubber boots.
6. Clean rags or disposable towels.
7. Absorbent material to soak up the spilled pesticide. Use either commercial spill control products or a material such as kitty litter, vermiculite, or sand.
8. A small shovel or dustpan to spread the absorbent material and to pick it up after.

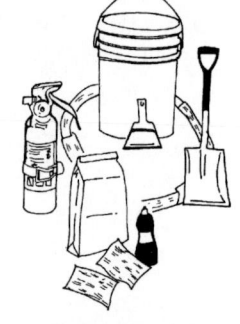

If you don't have a commercial spill control kit, put your own together

9. Heavy-duty plastic zip-lock bags to hold contaminated clothing or contaminated absorbent material..
10. The phone numbers of spill information hotlines, nearest Poison Control Center, local hospitals, and local authorities such as the state fire marshal and the local emergency management agency.
11. Written spill control procedures.

Store your spill control materials in a plastic five-gallon bucket with lid. Label the bucket clearly with a waterproof marker. The bucket can also be used to hold contaminated materials until you can dispose of them.

Damaged Pesticide Container

Check the pesticide containers in your shop and in your vehicle regularly. If you find a pesticide container that is cracked, partially crushed, rusting, or looks corroded, don't wait until it's actually leaking. You need to use up that pesticide or transfer it to another acceptable container as soon as possible.

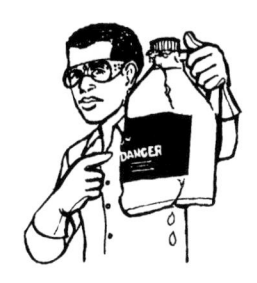

A leaky pesticide container requires immediate action

A more serious situation is a pesticide container that is *already* leaking. This demands immediate action. Put on any personal protective equipment, such as rubber gloves or goggles, that is required or suggested on the label.

If the leaking is severe, first contain the leak. A quick way to do this is to simply place the container inside a 5-gallon plastic bucket. If possible, turn the container so that the point of the leak is on top. Then take steps to transfer the pesticide. You have several options:

1. Transfer the pesticide into a spray tank and use it as soon as possible at an application site and rate that is listed on the label, or...
2. If you have another partially full container of the same product, transfer the pesticide to that container. Be sure that the second container holds exactly the same product at the same concentration and still has its label intact, or...
3. Transfer the pesticide to another clean, sturdy container that can be tightly closed. By law, a replacement pesticide container must be properly labeled. If possible, remove the label from the damaged container and securely attach it to the replacement container. Otherwise, mark the replacement

container with the product's name, EPA registration number, signal word, and percent concentration. Then get a copy of the label as soon as possible from your files, your pesticide supplier, or from the manufacturer (whose phone number is usually on the label), or...

4. Place the entire damaged container with its contents into a suitable larger container, such as a plastic bucket with lid. This should be only a short-term solution for liquid pesticides, however, since the label on a leaking container may become unreadable. The pesticide becomes useless unless you know what it is and can read the label directions. A leaking container of dry pesticide (granules or dust) can be placed inside a heavy duty plastic bag.
5. Meanwhile, salvage any puddled concentrate that you can (using a dust pan, sponge, or whatever), and then use kitty litter, sand, or a spill control product to soak up the rest for disposal. Check with the manufacturer to find out how best to decontaminate any leftover residue.
6. Remember to triple-rinse the damaged, empty container before disposal.

...temporarily place the leaky container in a bucket

Note: The contents of a leaky aerosol or other pressurized container can't be transferred to a replacement container and will have to be carefully disposed of according to label directions.

Replacing a Damaged Hose

A cracked hose on a termite rig or other high-pressure pumping unit demands replacement. Attaching the new hose correctly can prevent leaks and provide you with a stronger, longer-lasting coupling. Here are some tips:

- Release pressure from the old hose.
- Don't try to cut a hose held in your hand; place it firmly on a bench or other support. Wet the knife blade and cut the hose squarely.
- Lubricate the hose and coupling shank (hose barb) with soap and water. Oil should be used only on oil-resistant hoses.
- On especially tight connections you might want to countersink the inside of the hose slightly... don't alter the shank of the male coupling.

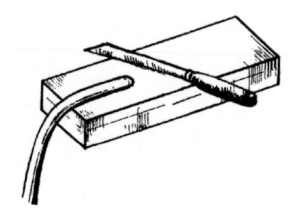

Place hose firmly on a support before cutting

- Keep the hose and the shank of the male coupling in alignment as you press them together. You may need to place the coupling in a vise for support. The hose should slide all the way to the base of the coupling shank.

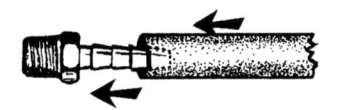

Slide hose all the way to the base of the coupling shank; soapy water will help it slide

- Place the clamp (or clamps) midway up the length of the shank making sure that the entire clamp is over the shank. Tighten it securely. Seal the end of the hose with rubber cement or shellac.

For emergency repairs in the field, it's a good idea to carry a short length of hose, some hose clamps, and two hose splice couplings. Then, if the hose cracks in the middle of a job, you can cut out and replace the cracked section. But remember to replace the entire hose as soon as possible, since a hose that has cracked in one place has weakened and is likely to crack again.

To prevent leaks from hoses in the first place, routinely inspect all hoses on termite rigs, sprayers, and dusters before you use them for the first time each day. This is also a good time to wipe down the hoses to remove any pesticide residue.

Key Points to Remember—Spills

- √ **Large leaks or spills require specially trained and equipped emergency crews.**
- √ **In a spill emergency, remember the three C's...Control, Contain, Clean up.**
- √ **Before you get near a pesticide spill, put on the appropriate personal protective equipment.**
- √ **Immediately block or redirect any spill that is moving towards ponds, streams, or sewers.**
- √ **A pest control service vehicle should carry a special spill control kit to clean up a pesticide spill.**
- √ **Many local and state authorities require that you report a pesticide spill over a certain size.**
- √ **As soon as the spill is under control, call your office or supervisor and explain the situation.**
- √ **To quickly contain the leak from a damaged pesticide container, temporarily place it inside a plastic bucket.**

STINGING AND VENOMOUS PESTS

Pest control work often puts technicians up against insects, spiders, scorpions, snakes, and things that can sting or inject venom. Some are dangerous, others merely painful. Regardless, you want to avoid being bitten or stung, and you need to know first aid measures to reduce pain, injury, or illness.

Bees and Wasps

Controlling bees and wasps can be interesting, but requires common sense and a certain amount of planning to avoid getting stung. If you suspect you might be allergic to bee or wasp stings, don't do this kind of work! A normal, nonallergic reaction to a sting is intense, immediate pain at the site of the sting, followed by localized swelling, warmth, and redness. These symptoms usually subside after a few hours but itching at the sting site may continue for days.

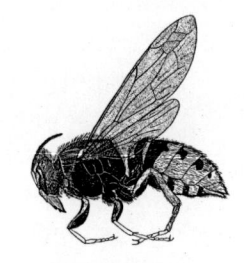

To avoid stings, plan wasp and bee control carefully

If you're stung on one part of your body and have a reaction in another part of your body, or a reaction beyond the first joint nearest the sting, you should be concerned. For example if you're stung on the foot and your entire leg swells up, or your face swells, or you break out in hives, you should see a physician. This may be an indication that your next sting could result in a life-threatening, allergic reaction leading to anaphylactic shock.

> *Symptoms of Anaphylactic Shock*
> - Itchy/hot palms or feet
> - Nausea, vomiting
> - Lumpy welts (hives) all over the body
> - Anxiety and feeling of impending doom
> - Headache
> - Breathing problems
>
>   —see discussion in *Allergy*

Precautions Around Bees and Wasps

The number one piece of advice given by pest control technicians who do stinging insect control is, "You have to be able to remain calm when the situation gets tense." Here are some practical tips to make control of stinging insects a painless experience:

- Avoid smelling like a flower--do not wear scented colognes or perfumes, or use scented soaps.
- Avoid looking like a flower--no brightly-colored clothing; no dark colors either (they think you're a bear attacking the nest. Honest!) White or light tan is best.
- For larger nests, cover your entire body--a bee suit with hood and veil is your best protection. Coveralls made of nylon or a slick, tight-weave fabric are a good second choice, along with gloves and a hat.
- Inspect the site before you begin. Note the location of overhead power lines if you're using a ladder or bee pole. Plan an escape route in case a quick getaway is necessary.
- Move quietly, slowly, and deliberately. Avoid vibrating the nest, making noise, or shining a light or casting a shadow on the nest.
- Be especially careful (and well-protected) if you go up on a ladder. When things go wrong on a ladder, there's no where to go but straight down!
- Have a can of a quick-freeze wasp spray handy on your person, not back in your vehicle.
- If a bee or wasp lands on your body, gently brush it off. If you're stung, cover your nose and mouth, protect your eyes, and quickly, but calmly, get away from the area (but see box below). The sting venom contains a pheromone that attracts other stinging insects to you. Wash the sting area to remove attractant.

Avoid vibrating the nest, making noise, or lights and shadows on the nest

If Attacked by Africanized Bees

- If attacked, cover your head with a shirt or cloth and RUN for shelter
- Africanized bees tend to target the eyes, ears, nose and mouth
- Don't flail your arms and try to swat the bees
- Don't jump in the water; the bees will just wait for you to surface
- Get away from the bees by going inside a building or car
- If you can't get indoors, run in a zigzag pattern until the bees disperse (they usually won't follow for more than 1/4 mile)
- If a victim is unable to escape, cover him with a blanket or tarp

First Aid for Bee and Wasp Stings

When a honey bee stings, it leaves behind its stinger with the venom sac attached. The stinger can continue to pump venom into the wound. In the past, experts advised that you remove the stinger by scraping it off since pinching it could inject more venom.

Now entomologists say that it doesn't matter how you get the stinger out. Apparently pinching the stinger and pulling it out doesn't release any more venom than if you scrape the stinger off. They discovered that the bee's stinger doesn't work like a bulb syringe after all. It's more like a pump and valve system and squeezing it doesn't force out more venom.

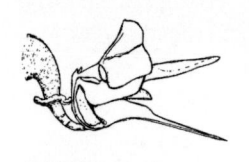

The longer a honey bee barbed stinger remains in the skin, the more venom is injected

But the longer the stinger remains in the skin, the more venom is released, and the larger the welt left by the sting. So, the experts say, use whatever method you like, but get that stinger out quickly. This advice applies only to bee stings. Yellowjackets and other wasps do not leave their stingers in your skin so, unfortunately, they can sting you again.

- Remove the stinger (in the case of a honey bee).
- Wash with soap and water (to remove any venom on skin surface).
- Put ice on the site to reduce the initial pain and minimize swelling.
- Analgesic, antihistamine, and cortisone creams may reduce pain and itch symptoms.
- If swelling extends beyond the sting site, or you notice any signs of an allergic reaction, see a physician (for more information, see *Allergy*).

Fire Ants

The fire ant's greatest impact on people is its sting. A single ant can sting repeatedly and a person is usually stung by many fire ants all at once. The initial pain is soon followed by pustules that itch and often leave scars. About 1% of the population is allergic to fire ant stings, with reactions ranging from severe swelling to respiratory and heart failure (see *Allergy*).

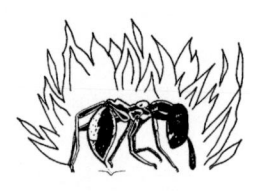

A single ant can sting repeatedly, leaving pustules that itch and often leaving scars

Precautions Around Fire Ants

If you work in fire ant areas, stay alert for ant mounds and foraging fire ants. When inspecting for fire ants, use a hand rake to pull back mulch, and use a screwdriver or other tool to turn over logs, stones, etc. rather than using your hands. Wear your pants tucked into or taped over a pair of boots.... a few dozen fire ants scrambling up inside your pants leg can ruin your day!

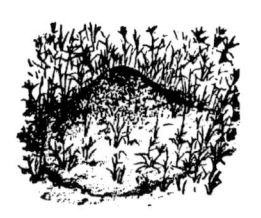

Keep an eye out for fire ant mounds!

First Aid for Fire Ant Stings

Same first aid as for bee and wasp stings.

Stinging Caterpillars

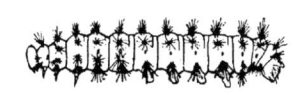

A number of moth caterpillars have what are called urticating hairs, designed to protect them from their natural enemies. The hairs are actually sharply pointed spines, sometimes with a poison gland at the base. When touched, the hairs break off and the poison is injected, causing inflammation of the skin and a burning sensation which may feel much like a bee sting or a nettle sting. There is often a delayed rash. In rare cases, inflammation can spread and the surrounding area can swell. The reaction can be more severe if the eyes, nose, or mouth are affected. (Young children may experience fever, nausea, and other symptoms.) Symptoms often persist for several days.

Fortunately, "stinging caterpillars" are uncommon around homes and yards. Most feed on native trees and shrubs and are found in wooded areas. Some of the more common stinging caterpillars are shown below.

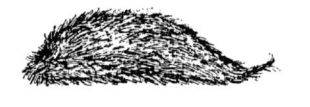

Puss caterpillar 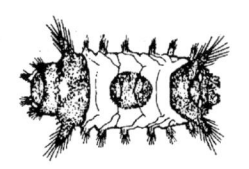   Saddleback caterpillar   Io moth caterpillar

The *puss caterpillar* is irresistibly furry; it begs to be petted. Sometimes people who pet it end up in the hospital. The puss caterpillar is found in the southeastern and south central states. It's about 1 inch long when fully-grown and is gray to reddish-brown in color.

The *saddleback caterpillar* is not fuzzy, but has a striking green "saddlecloth" on its back with a purplish-brown "saddle" in the middle... and bristly, irritating spines.

The *io moth caterpillar* is large and striking when fully-grown (about $2^1/_2$ inches). It is bright green with red and white stripes and four rows of short, stinging spines.

The caterpillar does not have to be alive to be able to sting; in fact, dry hairs from dead caterpillars appear to puncture the skin more easily. Even the hairs of common caterpillars, such as gypsy moth, can cause skin rashes in sensitive people. The caterpillars don't have to be handled for irritation to occur. The hairs may come from cocoons or be blown by the wind.

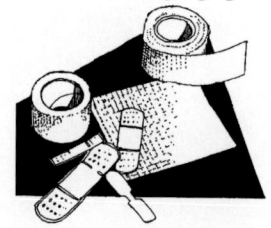

Spines can be pulled out with adhesive tape or a Band-Aid®

First Aid for Caterpillar Stings

First aid treatments are only partially effective at reducing the pain from the stings of these caterpillars, but may ease the itching and irritation.

- Wash the sting site with soap and water.
- Apply adhesive tape or a Band-Aid® and then remove it to pull out broken spines.
- Apply ice to reduce pain and swelling.
- Try antihistamine creams or other anti-itch creams.
- Seek medical attention if you have significant swelling or any severe or systemic symptoms.

Velvet Ants

Velvet ants get noticed. If you've ever seen one, you'll remember it. Their bodies are dark but they're covered with bright red, orange, white, or yellow velvety hairs. A velvet ant (also called a Mutillid) looks like a large fuzzy ant (up to 1 inch long), but isn't really an ant at all. The female velvet ant is a wingless wasp. She has long legs and can run rapidly. The male has wings but he's rarely seen.

Velvet ants are most common in the southern and western U.S. They're found outdoors, mostly in dry, open, sandy areas. The female lays her eggs in the nests of ground-nesting bees and wasps. Her larvae feed on the pupae of those bees or wasps.

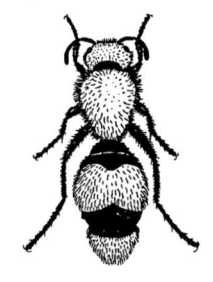

You usually only see one velvet ant at a time. But you may find large numbers where there have been large colonies of ground-nesting bees. Velvet ants may wander into homes during the summer months. Although they look cuddly, don't pick one up. The sting of a velvet ant is very painful. People are most often stung when they step on a velvet ant while barefoot.

Velvet ants are fuzzy and brightly colored

Velvet ants produce a squeaking sound when disturbed. That, combined with their bright coloration, serves as a warning to predators and people.

First Aid for Velvet Ant Stings

- Acute pain should only last about 30 minutes.
- Wash the sting area with soap and water and then apply ice to reduce the pain.
- If the pain continues, try applying a paste of baking soda and water, or use an analgesic, cortisone, or related pain-reducing cream.
- Seek medical attention if you have significant swelling or any severe or systemic symptoms.

Scorpions

When scorpions and people get together, the results can be painful, at the very least. The tail of the scorpion is equipped with a stout stinger, which injects venom. A scorpion often clasps the victim with its pincers and stings repeatedly. All stings are painful. The sting of a few scorpion species in the Southwest, California, and Mexico can be life-threatening. Children and older people, especially those with respiratory problems and heart disease, are most at risk.

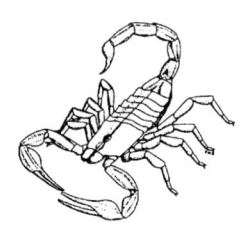

Stings of a few scorpion species are life-threatening

Pest Control Technician Safety Manual

Scorpions are not aggressive. They spend the day hidden under cover in burrows, under rocks and loose tree bark, in firewood, lumber piles, and debris, in outbuildings, in cracks and crevices in walls (especially rubble stone walls), in attics and suspended ceilings, under shake shingles, inside crawlspaces, under hot water heaters, and in other secluded places.

The sting causes a burning sensation at the sting site, usually with very little swelling or inflammation, but often with a positive "tap test," sharp pain when the site is tapped with a finger. Most scorpion stings are limited to the symptoms above, but systemic reaction may occur, although rarely, including hyperactivity, roving eyes, staggering gait, slurred speech, drooling, twitches, abdominal pain, and respiratory depression.

Precautions Around Scorpions

When inspecting in areas where scorpions are suspected or might occur, look out for scorpions, and wear long sleeves, long pants, socks, and gloves (heavy gloves if you are working in an area where some of the larger species occur). Avoid sticking an ungloved hand into dark places.

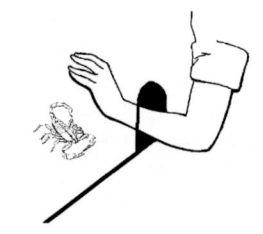

Do not stick an ungloved hand into a dark place!

First Aid for Scorpion Stings

- If a scorpion clasps on to you, remove it quickly to avoid multiple stings.
- Wash the bite site with soap and water.
- Apply ice to reduce pain and swelling.
- Elevate the bite site if possible.
- Capture the scorpion if possible (for identification).
- Seek medical attention (1) if the bite could have been from one of the dangerous species, or (2) if you have any significant swelling or systemic symptoms.

Spiders

Almost all spiders are venomous to some degree, but fortunately only a few are dangerous. Make a visit to your local zoo or museum. Find the reptile display and study the color patterns, features, and habitats of the poisonous snakes that occur in your region. These exceptions are various species of widow spiders (including the notorious black widow), brown spiders or "fiddleback" spiders (such as the brown recluse), the yellow sac spiders, and, in the Pacific Northwest, the hobo spider (formerly called the aggressive house spider).

The widows' venom is a neurotoxin that is immediately painful, and which can cause headache, dizziness, shortness of breath, profuse sweating, and often painful abdominal spasms and back pain. The bite can be fatal to children and adults in poor health.

Brown spiders and the hobo spider have a bite that is usually painless, followed by a localized burning or inflammation within an hour. A blister or blisters form, which can rupture and produce ulcerated sores with extensive tissue damage (necrosis) that may require surgery to repair. The bite of yellow sac spiders can cause similar reactions but usually to a much lesser degree.

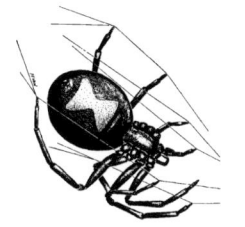

Black widow bites are immediately painful

Precautions Around Spiders

All of the spiders listed above except yellow sac spiders are shy and mostly found in hidden and dark areas. When inspecting in areas where these spiders are suspected or might occur, watch out for spiders, and wear long sleeves, long pants, socks, and gloves. Avoid sticking an ungloved hand into dark places. Look for the spiders' loose, irregular webs and cast skins and egg sacs. Check yourself periodically to make sure a spider isn't "hitchhiking" on your clothing.

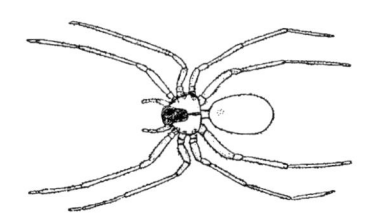

Brown recluse bites are painless but may produce ulcerated sores

Pest Control Technician Safety Manual

> *First Aid for Spider Bites*
> - Wash the bite site with soap and water.
> - Apply ice to reduce pain and swelling.
> - Elevate the bite site if possible.
> - Capture the spider if possible (for identification).
> - Seek medical attention: (1) if the bite could have been from any of the dangerous spiders listed above, or (2) if symptoms persist.

Snakes

In your job, you may be asked to control snakes, or you may encounter a snake while looking for mice or other pests. Can you be sure that snake is nonpoisonous? The only poisonous snakes found in the U.S. are rattlesnakes, copperheads, cottonmouths (water moccasins), and coral snakes. The first three are pit vipers. There are three ways to tell a pit viper from a nonpoisonous snake:

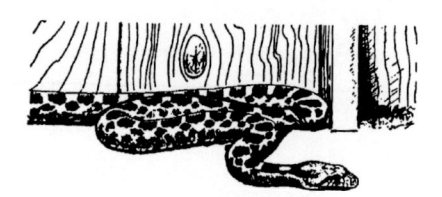

Poisonous snakes in the U.S. are rattlesnakes, copperheads, cottonmouths, and coral snakes

(1) A pit viper has a deep pit on each side of the head between the eye and the nostril. A nonpoisonous snake does not have a pit.

(2) The scales on the underside of a pit viper's tail are one row across. Rattlesnakes also have a "rattle" at the tip of the tail. The scales beneath the tail of a nonpoisonous snake are in two rows. *(You have to be good to check under a live snake's tail without being bitten! Fortunately, you can also see these characteristics in the shed skin of a snake.)*

(3) The dark pupil of the eye of a pit viper is vertically egg-shaped or elliptical. In bright light, it may be almost a closed slit. The pupil of a nonpoisonous snake is round. (Warning: A coral snake also has a round pupil.)

While the poisonous coral snake is not a pit viper, its bright color pattern is distinctive. It is ringed with black, plus red and yellow rings that are touching. Nonpoisonous mimics of the coral snake (like the scarlet king snake) have red and yellow rings separated by black. You can remember the difference with the saying, "Red on yellow, kill a fellow; red on black, friend of Jack."

Pit Viper   **Nonpoisonous Snake**

elliptical pupil   *round pupil*

deep pit

tail scales in one row   *tail scales in two rows*

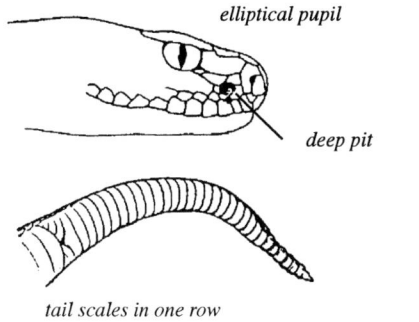

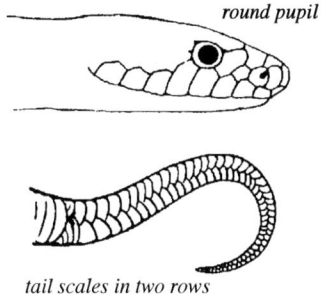

You can tell a poisonous pit viper from a nonpoisonous snake by its pits, tail scales, and pupils

Precautions Around Snakes

Wear long, loose pants, calf-high leather boots, and snake guards if working in rattlesnake areas. For snakes in high grass, sweep the grass with a long stick as you walk. Do not reach into hidden areas where there might be a snake without animal-handling gloves.

Be cautious when handling dead poisonous snakes. First of all, the snake may not be dead. For rattlesnakes, at least, the strike reflex remains active for up to one hour after they are dead, or even decapitated. Snake bites from dead rattlesnakes are surprisingly common. You can also get poisoned by scratching yourself on the fangs of a dead snake, even a long dead snake.

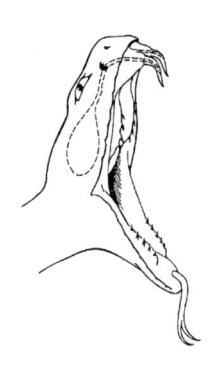

A rattlesnake strike reflex remains active for up to one hour after it is dead!

How to Catch a Snake, Poisonous or Otherwise

Especially if you are capturing a <u>poisonous</u> snake, use snake tongs or a snake hook, snake bag or cage, and wear leather boots and animal-handling gloves. A single snake, even a poisonous one such as a copperhead or rattlesnake, is not such a big problem, as long as you know where the snake is located and if it is easily accessible.

In these cases, it is usually a simple matter to pick up the snake with a snake hook or snake tongs and drop it into a plastic tub or other secure container. With a hook, just slip it under the snake about 1/3 back from the head and gently raise it off the ground. Slow and gentle works better than madly swiping at the snake.

With snake tongs, use the tongs to pin the snake's head to the ground so that it can be safely picked up just behind the head. Don't apply too much pressure or you can injure the snake's spine (assuming you are planning a release). Once restrained, and assuming you have the confidence and courage, pick it up just behind the jaws with your thumb and forefinger and support the rest of its body with your other hand. Place the snake into a garbage can with lid or a cage for transport and relocation.

If the snake is inside a building, but you don't know exactly where, or you know where but can't reach it, you can trap the snake by tacking several rat-size glue boards to a 16"x24" plywood sheet, or by using a commercial snake trap. Place glue traps up against a wall.

Another method is to use a pile of damp burlap bags or towels in a corner. After a couple of days, lift the entire pile with a shovel and drop into a plastic tub. If you're lucky, it will contain a snake!

First Aid for a Poisonous Snake Bite

The bite of a poisonous snake is always a medical emergency. Take the following steps if you are bitten:

- Stay calm and warm.
- Clean the bite, and let it bleed.
- Remove all rings, bracelets, watches, and constrictive clothing (there may be serious swelling).
- Hold the bitten area just below the heart, if possible, and keep it still.
- DON'T try to cut into the bite, suck out the venom, use a tourniquet, or apply ice.
- Get to a hospital or poison control center for treatment with the specific antivenin as soon as possible, or call 911.

Key Points to Remember—Stinging & Venomous Pests

- √ *When controlling social wasps and bees, avoid vibrating the nest, making noise, or shining a light or casting a shadow on the nest.*
- √ *Be especially careful (and well-protected) if you go up on a ladder to control bees or wasps.*
- √ *Have a can of a quick-freeze wasp spray handy on your person whenever inspecting or treating bees or wasps.*
- √ *When a honey bee stings you, get the stinger out quickly.*
- √ *When inspecting for fire ants, use a hand rake, not your hands, to pull back mulch, and use a screwdriver or other tool to turn over logs, stones, etc.*
- √ *When inspecting in hidden or dark areas, do not stick an unprotected hand into areas you can't see.*
- √ *If a scorpion clasps onto you, remove it quickly to avoid multiple stings.*
- √ *If bitten by a poisonous snake, get medical help. Don't try to cut into the bite, suck out the venom, use a tourniquet, or apply ice.*

STRESS

Why is stress discussed in a safety manual? Because job stress can lead to poor health and even injury. Job stress is real, not imaginary. Stress is the body's programmed response to danger or challenge. Sometimes called "fight or flight," this response helps us to better defend ourselves in a threatening situation. Short-term stress is beneficial: the nervous system

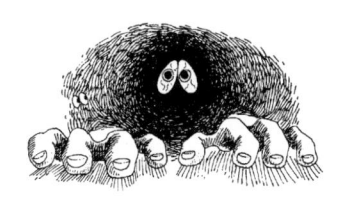

Job stress can lead to health problems and even increase your risk of injury

is aroused and the senses sharpened. Long-term stress keeps the body constantly on alert, which increases wear and tear to biological systems as all systems become fatigued. Medical research shows that long-term job stress can lead to cardiovascular disease, back and neck problems, depression and "burnout," and can contribute to unsafe work practices that lead to injuries.

Not all job stress is bad. Challenging work is energizing both physically and psychologically. However, you can become unacceptably stressed on the job when the requirements of your job consistently do not meet your capabilities, resources, or needs. About 40 percent of workers report their job is "very or extremely stressful," and 26 percent report they are "often or very often burned out or stressed by their work."

Stress Management

How do you deal with stress? Each person and company will be different, but here are a few recommendations:

- **Identify stress symptoms.** Early warning signs of excessive stress include headaches, sleep disturbances, difficulty in concentrating, short temper, upset stomach, job dissatisfaction, and low morale.
- **Learn what stress is.** Go to the library, look on the Internet. It is very important for you to realize that stress is a biological process that triggers certain reactions in your body. The same stressful working conditions would generate the same reactions in most other people.
- **Identify the job conditions causing your stress.** Specific job conditions that may lead to stress for some pest control technicians include the following:

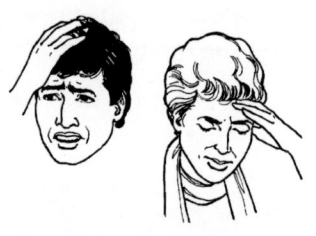

Signs of stress include headaches, short temper, and sleep disturbance

  • Heavy workload; no time for family, friends, and self
  • Not enough time between stops on route work
  • Shift work
  • No control of work; hectic and routine tasks
  • Conflicts with supervisors or coworkers
  • Customers with unrealistic expectations
  • Uncooperative customers
  • Rapid changes in job without training/preparation
  • Conflicting job expectations
  • Too many "hats to wear"
  • Low pay and job insecurity
  • Lack of opportunity for growth, advancement, or promotion

- Unpleasant working conditions
- Concerns about pesticide exposure
- Unfriendly work environment
- Consumer complaints

♦ **Talk to your supervisor or company management.** Group discussions between management and employees can identify and remedy stress problems in a small company, lead to better working conditions, and increase everyone's productivity.

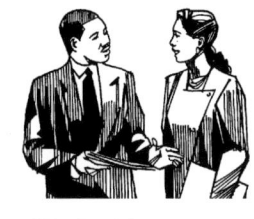

Work with managers to help reduce your job stress

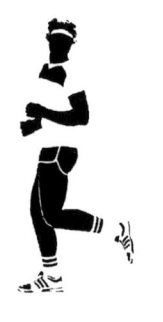

♦ **Reduce stress.** Correct or improve any stressful parts of your job that you have control over.

♦ **Manage your stress.** Different things work best for different people. Personal stress management tactics include creating a reasonable balance between work and family or personal life, better time management, and relaxation exercises. Regular exercise helps. For one thing, physically fit and healthy people find it easier to manage stress than those who are not. Besides burning off calories, exercise helps burn off frustration with conditions on the job. Group sports, such as basketball, softball, bowling, even golf, add the benefit of social interaction.

Exercise makes it easier to manage stress

Key Points to Remember—Stress

√ *Long-term job stress can lead to disease, injury, depression and "burnout."*

√ *Stress is a biological process that triggers the same reactions in almost everyone.*

√ *Physically fit and healthy people find it easier to manage stress than those who are not.*

√ *Group discussions between management and employees can identify and remedy stressful situations.*

√ *Work to correct or improve any stressful parts of your job.*

TETANUS

Lockjaw or tetanus is an acute, often fatal disease caused by bacteria that occurs in soil. Once it was common for people to die from lockjaw. It was a common cause of death for wounded soldiers in the Civil War. A victim of tetanus would have painful contractions and spasms of the voluntary muscles, including those of the jaw ("lockjaw"), ending in convulsive seizures. The first symptoms would be restlessness, headache, fever, difficulty in swallowing, and a sore jaw.

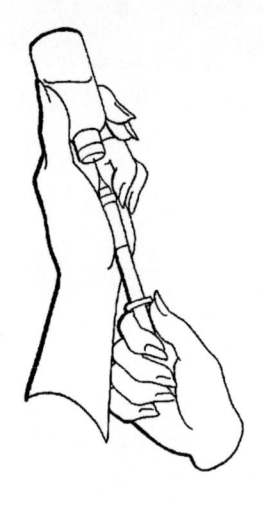

The bacteria can enter the body not only through a puncture wound (stepping on a nail), which everyone knows about, but also through a traumatic injury, scratch, burn, tear, frostbite, and even an animal scratch or bite (see *Wildlife* and *Attics and Crawlspaces*).

Tetanus is still around, even though we have a very successful vaccine. Make sure you have a booster tetanus shot every ten years (see *Vaccinations*). Even if you have had a tetanus shot within the last ten years, you may need a booster shot if you get a deep or contaminated wound. It is a physician's judgement call, so make sure you get medical advice. If you are approaching 50 years of age, or over 50, you should know that physicians recommend an adult immunization evaluation at age 50, since 70 percent of tetanus infections occur after that age.

Get a booster tetanus shot every 10 years

Key Points to Remember—Tetanus

√ **Lockjaw or tetanus is an acute, often fatal disease caused by bacteria that occurs in soil.**

√ **Get a booster tetanus shot every ten years.**

√ **If you are approaching 50 years of age, or over 50, check with your physician about a booster tetanus shot.**

TICK-TRANSMITTED DISEASES

Many diseases are transmitted by ticks to wildlife, livestock, domestic animals, and even people (see chart for tick-transmitted diseases in U.S.). This section addresses the three most important tick-transmitted diseases in the United States: Lyme disease, Rocky Mountain spotted fever, and ehrlichiosis.

Tick-Transmitted Human Diseases

Disease	Disease organism	Vector
Babesiosis	malaria-like parasite	*Ixodes scapularis*
Colorado tick fever	dengue-like virus	*Dermacentor andersoni*
Ehrlichiosis	bacterium	*Amblyomma americanum, I. scapularis*
Lyme disease	spirochete	*I. scapularis*
Q fever	rickettsia	*D. andersoni, A. americanum*, others
Relapsing fever	spirochete	*Ornithodoros* spp.
Rocky Mountain spotted fever	rickettsia	*D. andersoni, D. variabilis*
Tick paralysis	none, caused by toxin	*A. americanum, A. maculatum, D. andersoni, D. variabilis*
Tularemia	bacterium	*Dermacentor* spp., *Amblyomma* spp.

Lyme Disease

Lyme disease is the most common tick-transmitted disease in the U.S. The Centers for Disease Control (CDC) reported about 24,000 confirmed cases in 43 states and the District of Columbia for 2002. Lyme disease is most common along the Atlantic seaboard, the Great Lakes region, and in northern California.

Lyme disease is spread by the bite of an *Ixodes* tick, most commonly the black-legged tick (*Ixodes scapularis*). In areas where Lyme disease is common, up to 40 percent of the blacklegged ticks are infected. The tick larvae and nymphs normally pick up the infection when they feed on the white-footed mouse. The adult tick commonly feeds on the white-tailed deer. But any one of the tick life stages can attach to a person and pass on the disease organism.

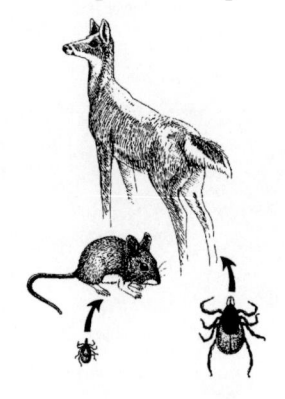

Blacklegged ticks and their mouse and deer hosts are common at wood edges

Symptoms of Lyme disease include the characteristic circular red rash at the bite site (in about 50 percent of cases) and flu-like symptoms. If untreated, these symptoms typically go away, but secondary symptoms appear weeks or months later. Migraine headaches, arthritis, and heart symptoms (weakness, dizziness, irregular heartbeat) can be the result of untreated Lyme disease. Early diagnosis is the key to successful treatment. Antibiotics can cure over 90 percent of cases treated within a few months of infection. If not caught early, treatment is more difficult. There may be long-term chronic symptoms and complications in a small percentage of these cases. Blood tests can determine if someone is infected.

A vaccine (Lymerix) designed to prevent Lyme disease in people at high risk was pulled off the market in 2002. There is currently no vaccine available.

Blacklegged ticks and their mouse and deer hosts are most common along edge habitats--woods bordered by an open grassy area. People living in homes on large wooded lots seem to be at highest risk. The ticks are active almost year-round, but the number of Lyme disease cases peaks in July.

Rocky Mountain Spotted Fever

Rocky Mountain spotted fever (RMSF) is a severe, acute infectious disease in humans caused by the microorganism *Rickettsia rickettsii*. Symptoms include the following:

- A fever that reaches 103° F.
- Severe headache, often unrelieved by aspirin or other painkillers
- Severe muscle and sometimes joint aches
- Nausea or vomiting in 60 percent of cases
- A rash on the ankles, soles, wrists, and palms that occurs two or more days after the onset of the illness

The rash resembles the measles, and is the primary means of diagnosis. Unfortunately, some rashes appear late or not at all, and then diagnosis is very difficult. Mortality is 20-25 percent when the disease is untreated with antibiotics.

The disease occurs throughout the U.S. but, despite its name, most cases occur in the east from Maryland south to the Carolinas. RMSF is vectored by a number of ticks including the Rocky Mountain wood tick (*Dermacentor andersoni*) in the Rocky Mountain states, and the American dog tick (*Dermacentor variabilis*) in the eastern two-thirds of the country and the west coast. The tick must remain attached for more than two hours (some sources say six to ten hours) in order to transmit the disease.

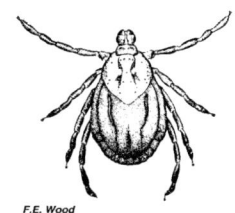

The American dog tick must remain attached for more than two hours to transmit RMSF

Illustration F.E. Wood

Ehrlichiosis

Ehrlichiosis (pronounced ur-lik-ee-OH-sis) is a rickettsial disease named after *Ehrlichia*, the genus of the bacteria that causes it. The first time the disease was diagnosed in the U.S. was in 1987.

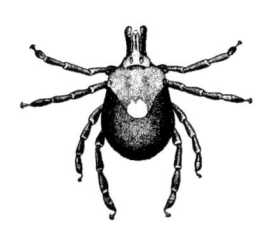

Ehrlichiosis symptoms appear about seven days after the bite of the lone star tick

Illustration F.E. Wood

Researchers have identified five types of ehrlichiosis attacking dogs, horses, sheep, and cattle, and two, or perhaps three, attacking people. The two primary human ehrlichioses are transmitted by the lone star tick (*Amblyomma americanum*) in the south central and southeastern U.S., and the blacklegged tick (*Ixodes scapularis*) in the upper midwest and the northeast. From 1986 through 1997, the Centers for Disease Control confirmed over 1200 cases. Many more cases have probably gone unreported because the symptoms of ehrlichiosis mimic other diseases including Lyme disease, Rocky Mountain spotted fever (RMSF), and the flu.

Most cases develop between April and September. Symptoms usually appear about seven days after the tick bite, but the range is 1-21 days. It appears that the majority of people who get ehrlichiosis have mild symptoms or no symptoms at all. When symptoms do appear, they are similar to those of RMSF. A rash is rare, but when it occurs it may resemble that of RMSF, although typically less prominent and more variable in appearance and location. For those who do develop symptoms, quick treatment with antibiotics (usually doxycycline) is important. If untreated, the disease organism invades white blood cells, affecting the immune system and reducing the body's ability to fight other infections. In the most severe cases, ehrlichiosis can cause kidney or respiratory failure, and there have been a number of deaths from the disease.

Tick Paralysis

Tick paralysis is a rare but potentially deadly condition that occurs while a tick is attached and feeding. The mechanics of the paralysis are not well understood. Researchers believe a toxin is released into the bloodstream by the tick, and then the toxin binds to fibers of nerves that control muscles. Tick paralysis can affect dogs, livestock, wildlife, and people, usually children.

Rocky Mountain wood ticks, lone star ticks, Gulf Coast ticks, and American dog ticks are known to cause tick paralysis. In most, if not all, cases an adult female tick must feed for at least five days near the head or neck. About a day before the onset of paralysis, the victim may feel irritable, tired, with some general undefined pain, and may have prickly, tingling sensations on the skin. The person then becomes uncoordinated, and the legs are slowly paralyzed. The paralysis ascends up to the arms, neck, and face, and may reach the muscles needed for breathing. The symptoms of advanced tick paralysis are very similar to polio, and the death rate can be as high as 12 percent.

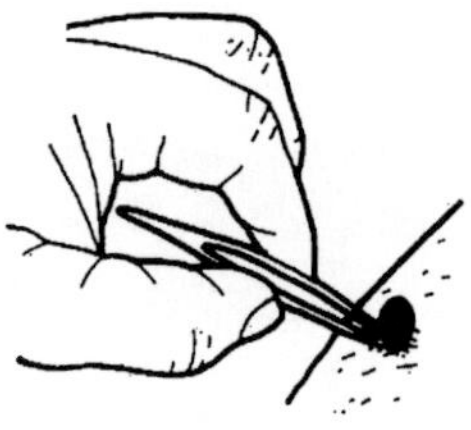

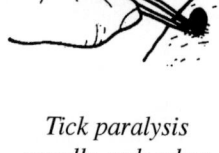

If the tick drops off naturally or is removed manually before the paralysis is too far along, the patient usually recovers completely, sometimes within a few hours. The key treatment for tick paralysis is to find and remove the tick.

Tick paralysis usually ends when the tick is removed

If you experience a loss of coordination or any type of paralysis, see a physician or go to an emergency room.

Precautions in Tick Areas

If you work outdoors in tick-infested areas:

- Avoid dense undergrowth and long grass or weeds.
- Wear long sleeves and long pants. Light-colored clothing helps you see ticks. Tuck pants legs into your socks and boots, and keep your collar buttoned.
- Use wide masking tape to tape your socks to your pants and tape your sleeves to your wrists. The idea is to eliminate any gaps that allow ticks to crawl up under clothing.

- Spray shoes, clothing, and exposed skin with an insect repellent that contains DEET (diethyltoluamide). Tick repellents containing permethrin are available in most states for use on clothing.
- Wear gloves if you're trapping or handling deer, white-footed mice, or other small mammals that may be hosts for ticks. Dispose of dead animals in plastic bags.
- Shower at the end of the workday and check yourself for ticks.
- If you are bitten by a tick, remove it immediately and save it in alcohol.
- If you become sick within two weeks after being exposed to ticks, or you get a rash, or experience a loss of coordination or partial paralysis, see a physician immediately.

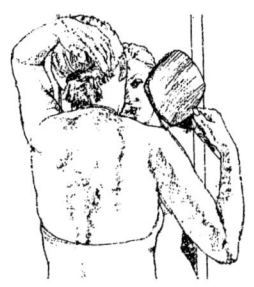

Shower and check yourself for ticks at the end of the workday

How to Remove a Tick

Remove the tick as soon as you discover it. Don't delay because the longer the tick is attached and feeding, the greater your chances of getting a tick-vectored disease like Lyme disease.

- Using blunt (not sharp, pointed) tweezers, grab the tick's head as close to the skin as you can. Pull slowly but steadily. Pull in the reverse of the direction in which the mouthparts are inserted. Don't twist as you pull, pull straight back. You don't want to break off the head or leave mouthparts in the skin. If any part of the tick remains in the skin, gently scrape it away.
- If you don't have tweezers available (they should, however, be part of your insect collection kit), don't remove the tick with bare hands. Use a tissue, cloth, or even a leaf to grab the tick.
- Don't squeeze, crush, or puncture the tick's body. You've seen guys puncture the tick with their thumb nail to kill it. Not a good idea because that releases the tick's bodily fluids which can contain disease organisms.
- Don't apply a hot match or cigarette to the tick or cover it with substances like Vaseline, nail polish, mineral oil, insect repellent, gasoline, etc. This

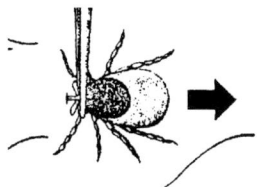

Grab the mouthparts of the tick close to the skin and pull straight outward

doesn't make the tick back out but instead can stress the tick and cause it to regurgitate more fluids into the bite.
- After removal, wash your hands, the bite area, and the tweezers with soap and water. Apply an antiseptic to the bite area.
- It's a good idea to place the tick in a small vial of alcohol in case you need to have it identified later.
- Check the bite area daily for any signs of infection or a bull's-eye rash. If you develop a rash anywhere on your body, flu-like symptoms, or any type of partial paralysis within two to four weeks after the bite, contact your physician.

Key Points to Remember—Tick-transmitted Diseases

- √ **The three most common tick-transmitted diseases are Lyme disease, Rocky Mountain spotted fever, and ehrlichiosis.**
- √ **A rash is a common symptom for Lyme disease, Rocky Mountain spotted fever, and sometimes ehrlichiosis.**
- √ **Blacklegged ticks are most common along edge habitats—woods bordered by an open grassy area.**
- √ **Protect yourself if you must work outdoors in tick-infested areas.**
- √ **If you are bitten by a tick, remove it immediately and save it in alcohol.**
- √ **If you become sick within two weeks after being exposed to ticks, or you get a rash, see your physician.**

TUBERCULOSIS (TB)

Tuberculosis, or TB, is the leading cause of death in the world due to an infectious agent. Once, there were TB hospitals or "sanitoriums" all over the U.S. Then antibiotics and other drugs were developed to control TB. Unfortunately, a resurgence of outbreaks in the United States is bringing new attention to TB. Immunosuppressed persons, particularly those infected with human immunodeficiency virus (HIV), are at highest risk. Drug-resistant strains of TB have contributed to the problem. Some outbreaks have involved the transmission of multidrug-resistant strains, which are often fatal. Outbreaks have occurred in hospitals, correctional institutions, homeless shelters, nursing homes, and residential care facilities for AIDS patients. Several hundred employees have become infected nationwide after workplace exposure to TB.

TB is carried in airborne particles which are generated by infected people when speaking, coughing, sneezing or when certain medical procedures are performed. The particles are so small that normal air ventilation keeps them airborne and circulates the particles throughout a room, building, or vehicle.

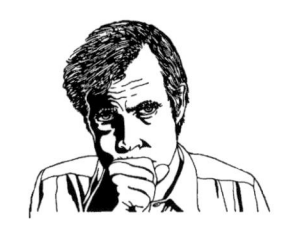

TB is carried in tiny airborne particles that float in the air

Workers most at risk are those working in hospitals, prisons, drug treatment centers, nursing homes, and homeless shelters. If you work in these types of accounts, you are at some degree of risk as well.

According to the Centers for Disease Control (CDC) guidelines, you must wear a NIOSH-approved high efficiency (HE) filtered respirator (or Class N-100, R-100 or P-100 respirator) if you enter a room occupied by someone with suspected or confirmed infectious TB. In medical facilities you may see a TB warning, a "STOP" sign, and "No Admittance Without Wearing A Type N100 or More Protective Respirator" or similar warning signs. Do not enter that room unless (1) you have proper authorization, (2) you are wearing the proper respirator, and (3) you have been trained in the use of that respirator.

Key Points to Remember—Tuberculosis

- √ **TB is carried in airborne particles which are generated by infected people when speaking, coughing, sneezing or when certain medical procedures are performed.**
- √ **TB particles are so small that normal air ventilation keeps them airborne and circulates the particles throughout a room, building, or vehicle.**
- √ **Do not enter a posted tuberculosis area without proper training, authorization, and any required protective equipment.**

VACCINATIONS

A pest control technician's work may increase the risks of certain diseases for which vaccines are available. You may, for example, work in health care facilities. Should you be vaccinated with hepatitis B vaccine or not? Such decisions are personal, made only after talking with your physician and your supervisor at work.

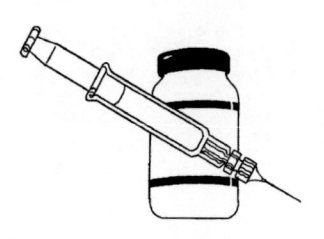

Should you be vaccinated for any of these diseases? Check with your physician

As with any medical procedure or medication, immunizations are associated with a risk of an adverse reaction. Typical reactions may include warmth, redness, and tenderness at the site of the injection. Potentially serious reactions vary according to the type of immunization and include the risk, though very rare, for seizures, damage to the brain or central nervous system, and death. However, most reactions are minor and treatable. There are so few deaths that could plausibly be connected to vaccine, and the risk is so small, that it is hard to assess statistically.

Listed below are the vaccines to control diseases that you might face in certain types of pest control work. The recommendations for when they should be given come from various sources at the Centers for Disease Control (CDC).

Hepatitis B Vaccine

Hepatitis B is a virus that is transmitted by infected blood (see *Bloodborne Pathogens*). The disease has a long incubation period and can cause severe or chronic liver disease. Medical workers and others with occupational risk of exposure to blood or blood-contaminated body fluids should be vaccinated. Technicians who regularly work in hospitals and other medical facilities, and who might be exposed to blood and other potential infectious materials, should consider vaccination. Also consider vaccination for hepatitis B if you have been trained and authorized to provide first aid in case of emergency.

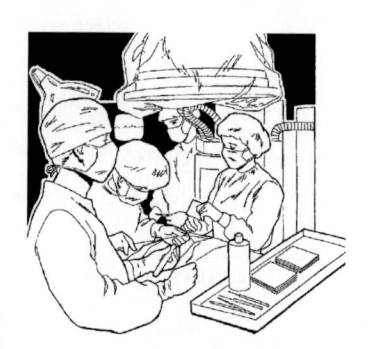

Consider hepatitis B vaccination if you often work in medical facilities

The vaccine is given in three doses: the second dose 1-2 months after the first, and third dose 4-6 months after the first.

Influenza Vaccine

Influenza, better known as the flu, is an acute viral respiratory disease that everyone is familiar with. It is highly contagious, spread by person-to-person contact and airborne droplet spray. Severe cases of flu can be dangerous, sometimes leading to pneumonia and, in rare cases, death.

Many different but related viruses cause influenza. A flu shot given at the beginning of flu season in the fall offers good, but not absolute, protection against flu over the next year or so. Flu shots in a given year contain a mix of those strains of influenza anticipated to cause problems during the coming flu season, but give little protection against unexpected strains of the virus. A flu shot is often combined with a vaccine effective against pneumonia.

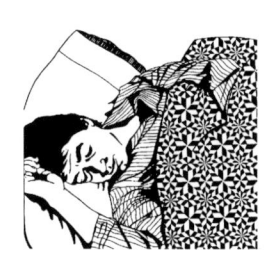

A flu shot provides protection from the flu for one year

In general, the following people should get flu shots:

- Adults 50 years of age and older.
- People with a high-risk of complications from flu.
- Any person over six months of age who wishes to reduce the likelihood of becoming ill with influenza. Many companies recommend that their employees get flu shots to reduce illness and time off of work.
- Care givers, household members, and other people who may infect high-risk persons. Examples include people working in hospitals, nursing homes, and chronic-care facilities who have contact with patients or residents. Whether a pest control technician should be considered in this category would depend on the degree of contact and interaction with patients and residents.

Lyme Disease Vaccine

A vaccine (Lymerix) designed to prevent Lyme disease in people at high risk was pulled off the market in 2002. A replacement vaccine is not available at this time.

Plague Vaccine

Primarily a bacterial disease of rats, ground squirrels, prairie dogs, and other rodents, as well as hares and rabbits, plague can be passed on to humans, usually through the bite of a flea (see discussion under *Rodents*). Most U.S. cases (about ten per year) involve people coming into contact with wild animals, especially ground squirrels, rabbits, and prairie dogs in the western states.

Pest Control Technician Safety Manual

Up until 1999, there was a plague vaccine that consisted of a series of three inoculations. Its effectiveness was questionable and the manufacturer stopped making it. A new vaccine is currently being tested for the military, but it will not be available until 2007 at the earliest.

Rabies Vaccine

An acute infectious disease of warmblooded animals, rabies is inevitably fatal if untreated (see discussion under *Wildlife*). Because rabies has a long incubation period, a series of rabies vaccinations can be given after a person has been bitten or scratched by a rabid animal, and will provide full protection as long as symptoms have not appeared before inoculation.

The vaccines can also be given as a preventative. The CDC suggests that you consider preventative vaccination if your work brings you in contact with potentially rabid dogs, cats, skunks, raccoons, bats, or other wildlife species. You would then get a booster dose every 2 years, or have a blood test to see if you need the booster dose.

Note: This preventative vaccination against rabies does NOT eliminate the need for additional therapy after exposure to rabies. It does, however, simplify postexposure treatment by eliminating the need for human rabies immune globulin (HRIG) injections and by decreasing the number of postexposure doses of vaccine needed.

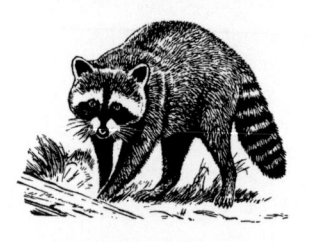

Consider a preventative rabies vaccine if you do a lot of animal control work

Tetanus Vaccine

Lockjaw or tetanus is an acute, often fatal disease caused by bacteria that occurs in soil (see *Tetanus*). All adults need a tetanus vaccination, which provides protection for at least ten years. Boosters are recommended at ten-year intervals. *You need a booster shot if it has been ten years since your last tetanus shot.* Physicians recommend an adult immunization evaluation at age 50, since 70 percent of tetanus infections occur after that age.

A clean, minor wound received less than ten years since your last tetanus shot will not usually require an additional tetanus booster. A booster is appropriate for serious wounds if you have not received a tetanus shot within the preceding five years.

Key Points to Remember—Vaccinations

- √ **Consider hepatitis B vaccination if you regularly work in medical facilities, or you are trained and authorized to perform first aid.**
- √ **A flu shot provides about one year's protection.**
- √ **All adults need a tetanus vaccination or booster, which lasts 10 years.**
- √ **There is a preventative rabies vaccine available for those whose work brings them in regular contact with potentially rabid animals.**

VIOLENCE

Workplace violence is an important safety issue in today's workplace. Its most extreme form, homicide, is the second leading cause of fatal occupational injury in the United States. On average, three workers die each day under violent circumstances. In addition, hundreds of thousands of workers are in some way physically assaulted on the job.

Today, risk of personal attacks on pest control technicians is a fact of life. You need to identify situations where violence could erupt, and act to avoid it. Examples of situations where you face sudden violence include the following:

- Servicing inner-city drug areas and gang territories, and being seen as an outsider
- Servicing violence-prone public housing, low-income apartments, and dangerous inner-city neighborhoods
- Collecting cash from customers
- Becoming caught up in arguments and grudges with coworkers or customers
- Getting involved in aggressive driving, traffic arguments, and road rage

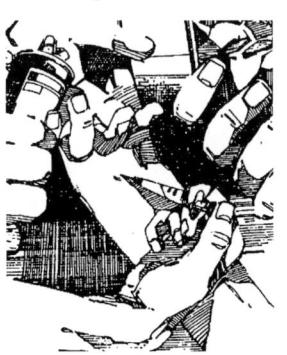

Be cautious in areas of illegal drug activity

Pest Control Technician Safety Manual

Precautions Against Violence

Safety precautions in violence-prone areas include common sense procedures such as the following:

- Stand to the side of a door after knocking (to avoid a bullet through the door).
- Clearly identify yourself before entering, and again once you are inside.
- Do not act in a threatening manner.
- Do not carry a pistol-style bait applicator so that it might be mistaken for a real gun.
- Do not look curious about what is going on around you, particularly if drugs or other illegal activities might be involved.
- When possible, have a well-known, recognizable employee of the property accompany you.
- Do not enter a building or residence if you believe you might face a significant risk of personal attack by entering. When in doubt, contact the site manager or your supervisor for advice.
- Drive gently (nowadays, traffic arguments sometimes end with a bullet).
- Be courteous and diplomatic with coworkers.
- Be willing to back down in a confrontation.

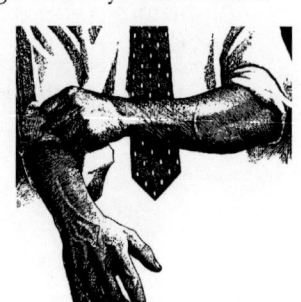

Be willing to back down in a confrontation

Key Points to Remember—Violence

√ **Identify situations where violence could erupt, and act to avoid it.**
√ **If you face a significant risk of personal attack by entering a building or residence, do not enter.**
√ **Drive gently to avoid road rage attack.**
√ **Back down in confrontations.**

WAREHOUSES

A warehouse is a busy place. Fast-paced activity during certain critical times often leads to injuries. Warehouses present many potential hazards such as unguarded drop-offs, improperly stacked materials, erratic forklifts, and hazardous materials. The fatal injury rate for the warehousing industry is higher than the national average for all industries.

Of course, certain areas or operations within a warehouse present greater hazards than others. According to the American Society of Safety Engineers, the following operations have historically contributed to significant numbers of injuries and are considered to be the most hazardous: docks, powered industrial trucks, conveyors, materials storage, manual lifting/handling and charging stations. Other serious problems include unsafe use of forklifts, improperly stacked products, unguarded floor or wall openings or holes, inadequate fire safety provisions, chemical exposure, improper use of lockout procedures, lack of ergonomics and failure to wear personal protective equipment.

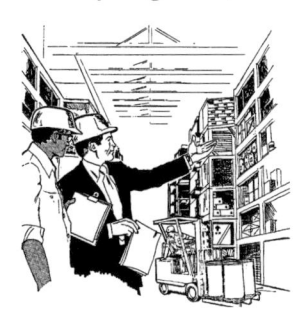

Fast paced activity in a warehouse often leads to injuries

The most common hazards facing pest control technicians working in warehouses are the following:

Unsafe Activity on Docks

According to the National Safety Council (NSC), injuries that occur at docks are responsible for 10 to 25 percent of all workplace injuries. Employees and visitors alike are at risk. When working at a loading dock--

- Keep clear of loading dock edges.
- Be aware that dock plates can be very slippery.
- Be careful when sharing a dock with a forklift or other moving equipment. You can be struck, knocked off the dock, or pinned, not only from the front, but from "rear-end swing."
- Don't engage in "dock jumping," which can lead to serious ankle, knee and back injuries. Use the stairs instead.

Forklifts, Hand Jacks, and Pallet Jacks

Some 100 employees are killed and 95,000 injured each year in accidents involving forklifts and other types of powered industrial trucks. These devices have a high center of gravity, turn more sharply than an auto (because its rear wheels do the steering) and may weigh three to four times more than an auto. All of these factors contribute to forklift tipover, which, according to OSHA statistics, is responsible for around one quarter of all fatal injuries to operators.

Pallet jacks or hand jacks (also called walkies), although far less massive, still pose some of the same hazards as forklifts.

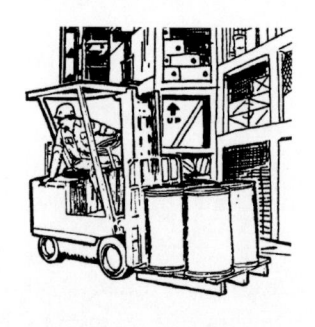

Watch for forklift traffic in crowded aisles and when approaching corners

Forklift, Hand Jack, and Pallet Jack Precautions

- Watch for forklift or pallet jack traffic in crowded aisles.
- Move slowly when approaching blind corners or doorways.
- Don't come between a working forklift and a wall or stack of products.
- Don't operate a forklift or pallet jack unless you are specifically trained to do so.

Improper Stacking of Products

OSHA found that almost 50% of all warehouse injuries occurred in the storage area. Technicians are often working in the aisles between stacked materials, especially when doing rodent work. Take the following precautions around stacked products:

- Look out for stacks that are too high or that are crooked and may fall.
- Be wary when working around obviously damaged or degraded pallets. Loads can fall from racking or storage if a pallet breaks.
- Move away when warehouse workers begin lifting palleted materials.
- When moving stored materials, remove one product at a time from shelves.
- Restack products with heavier loads on lower or middle shelves.

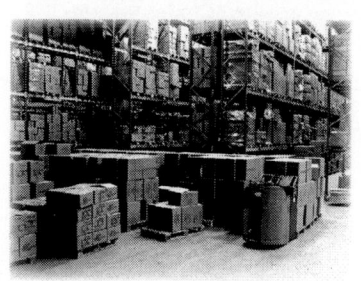

Look out for stacks that are too high or that are crooked and that could fall on you

Photo © Harald Tjøstheim/iStockphoto

- If you do move product, use proper lifting techniques. Bend at the knees, keep close to the load, and use the arms and legs to lift, and do not twist at the waist when turning with a load.

Failure to Use Proper Personal Protective Equipment

Chemical exposure and physical danger is not unusual in a warehouse. Chemical exposure can occur when a lift truck fork punctures a container holding solvent. Or a container of a toxic chemical may be damaged if dropped. Other exposures range from everyday use of chemicals to battery acid.

Physical dangers can include materials dropping down from above, heavy items pinching or crushing feet, plastic or metal bands that snap back when cut, and excessive noise.

A warehouse is responsible for ensuring the safety of its employees and its contractors and guests. Each warehouse will have rules on what personal protective equipment (PPE) is required for different jobs and different areas of the warehouse. The pest control company and its technicians must, in turn, follow the requirements of the warehouse.

Required PPE may include hard hats, gloves, steel-toed shoes, goggles, hearing protection, and respirators.

Improper Lockout/Tagout Procedures

Various machines, devices and operations in a warehouse have enough energy to cause serious injury to people. All warehouses must have a lockout/tagout program (LOTO) to prevent equipment from being accidentally turned on during service or maintenance. Examples include conveyors, forklifts, lift gates, automatic doors, elevators, and even small devices such as fans, battery chargers, and the like.

A pest control technician treating or working around a piece of equipment that could start up or release energy and cause injury is subject to the lockout/tagout rules of the warehouse. Do not remove lockout devices or tags or attempt to start the equipment.

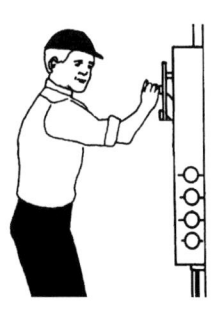

Never remove lockout devices or tags or attempt to start tagged equipment

For more information, see the detailed discussion at *Lockout/Tagout*.

Unsafe Handling of Hazardous Materials

Just as in pest control offices, chemicals are common in warehouses. Wear the proper personal protective equipment if you are handling chemicals in warehouses. Be alert to leaking product in storage.

Chemical exposure can also be from carbon monoxide produced from powered equipment or trailer trucks.. Make sure the area you're working in is adequately ventilated. If a carbon monoxide alarm goes off, leave the area immediately.

Key Points to Remember—Warehouses

- √ **Don't engage in "dock jumping," which can lead to serious ankle, knee and back injuries.**
- √ **Watch for forklift or pallet jack traffic in crowded aisles.**
- √ **Look out for stacks that are too high or that are crooked and may fall.**
- √ **Follow the PPE requirements of the warehouse**
- √ **Do not remove lockout devices or tags or attempt to start the equipment.**

WARNING SIGNS

Do not ignore safety warning signs. They are there because of some hazard to your life or health, or to the life and health of others in the area. Some warning signs mean you should not even enter the area without special training and authorization. Other signs indicate that you need to take certain precautions before entering or working in the area. If you are not sure what the signs mean, or what precautions you need to take, contact site management or your supervisor for guidance.

On the next pages are samples of signs commonly seen in commercial, medical, and industrial accounts. Review the signs to make sure you know if you can enter the area, or what precautions are necessary if you do.

Pest Control Technician Safety Manual

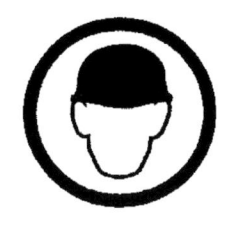

Hard hat area

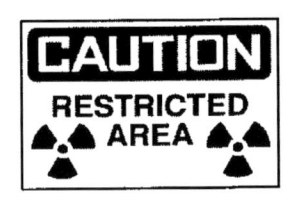

Restricted radiation area

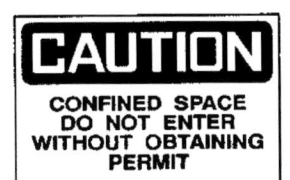

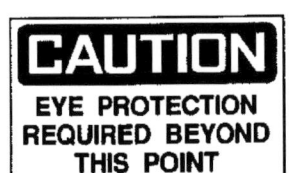

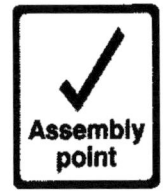

Assembly point for fire or other emergency

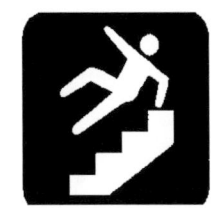

Fall hazard

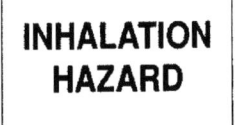

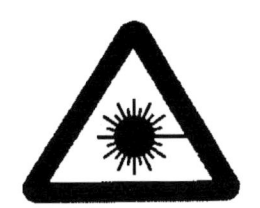

Laser equipment

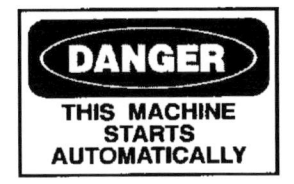

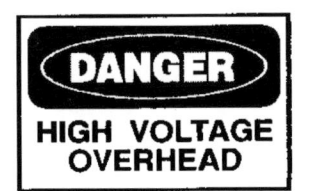

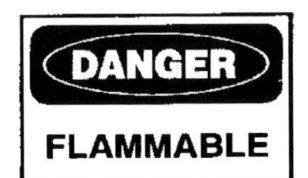

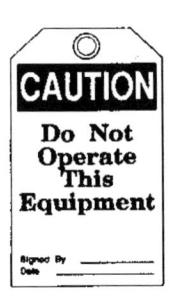

Tagout

| 205 |

Pest Control Technician Safety Manual

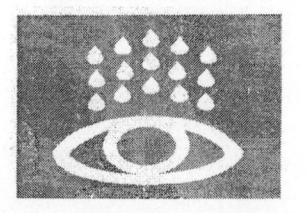

Eyewash station

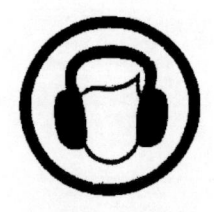

Hearing protection required

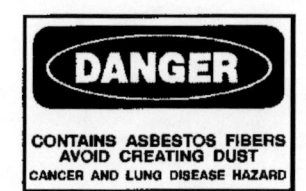

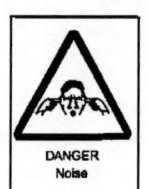

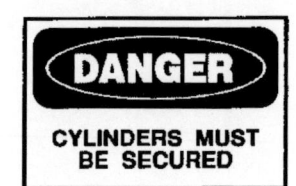

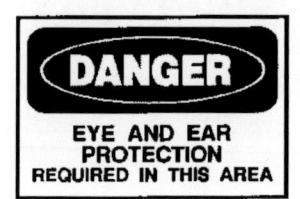

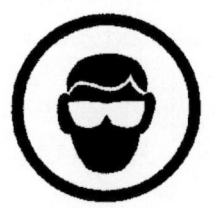

Eye protection required

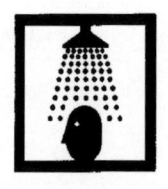

Emergency shower

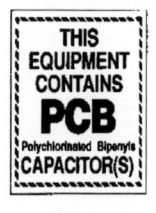

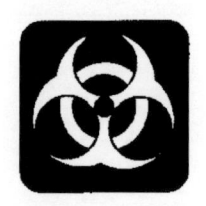

Biological hazards

WILDLIFE

Pest control technicians who do animal control face risk of bites and scratches from trapped or aggressive wildlife and feral animals (such as feral cats). Technicians also face risk of disease or ectoparasites (fleas, mites, ticks, etc.) that can be transmitted from those animals. (See also *Rodents*, *Hookworm*, and *Tick-transmitted Diseases*.)

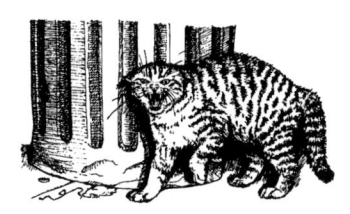

Use animal control equipment and gloves when capturing wild or feral animals

Rabies

After years of decline in the U.S., rabies is once again on the increase. Human deaths from rabies are still rare, however, since most people in the U.S. are treated if they are bitten by an animal known or suspected to be rabid.

There is no way to detect rabies in humans until symptoms appear. And almost no one survives once symptoms appear. (In 2004, a Wisconsin teenager contracted rabies from a bat bite and *became the first known person to survive rabies* despite not having received rabies vaccine prior to symptom onset.) If there's any chance that the animal was rabid, you <u>must</u> be vaccinated.

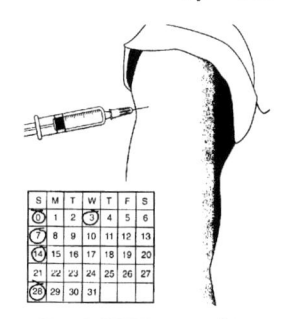

You MUST get rabies shots if you are bitten or scratched by a rabid animal

Fortunately, the rabies vaccine has been improved over the years. Instead of 21 shots in the stomach as in the old days, you now typically receive five shots in the arm over a period of 28 days. Today's vaccines are more effective and produce fewer side effects. For the most part, rabies vaccine is given only after exposure to the disease...after you've been bitten or scratched by an animal or exposed to its saliva. There is also a preventative vaccine sometimes given to those considered to be high-risk such as veterinarians, animal control officers and, in some cases, pest control technicians who trap wildlife where rabies is a problem (see *Vaccinations*).

How Can You Tell if an Animal Is Rabid?

Rabies can be contagious even <u>before</u> symptoms appear, so a healthy-looking animal can transmit the disease. Even a dead animal can transmit rabies if its saliva comes in contact with a cut or skin abrasion. When symptoms of rabies eventually appear in an infected animal, the symptoms can be extremely variable. Some animals exhibit *"furious rabies,"* meaning that they will attack anything that moves. Skunks, raccoons, foxes, ground hogs, and dogs are most likely to exhibit this aggressive form of rabies.

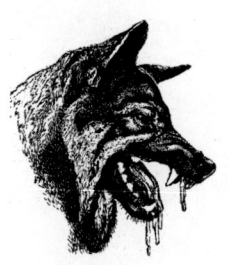

Other animals exhibit what is called *"dumb rabies."* They may appear to be unusually friendly, or may stumble or appear disoriented. Animals may stop eating or drinking. Bats may be found on the ground, unable to fly.

Rabies often involves some degree of paralysis in animals. Paralysis of throat muscles can cause an animal to drool, whine, or choke. Infected animals may make strange noises like chattering or screaming. Basically, if an animal is acting differently than you would expect it to, suspect rabies unless you can determine otherwise.

Some animals exhibit "furious rabies" and will attack anything that moves

Signs of Rabies in Animals

The main clue that an animal may be rabid is unusual behavior:

- A tame animal acting wild
- A wild animal acting unusually tame
- An animal acting extremely aggressive and excitable
- An animal that appears to be weak-limbed and lethargic, unable to raise its head
- An animal that is unable to make any sound or appears to be choking (neck and throat muscles may become paralyzed)

Because symptoms are so variable and because other conditions cause similar symptoms, you can't tell if an animal has rabies unless it is killed and the brain tissue tested. Distemper, toxoplasmosis, and poisoning from lead, mercury, or antifreeze can also cause an animal to exhibit some of these same symptoms.

It's often said that if nocturnal animals are active during the day when you don't expect to see them, you should suspect rabies. However, there are certain qualifiers.

Female raccoons, for example, may be active during the day when they are feeding young.

Likewise, shabby looking animals are not necessarily rabid. Nursing females sometimes look unkempt because the young pull at her fur as they nurse.

High-Risk Animals

Wild animals account for nine of ten rabies cases reported to the CDC. Raccoons continued to be the most frequently reported rabid wildlife species (37%), followed by skunks (31%), bats (17%), foxes (6%), and other wild animals, including rodents and lagomorphs [rabbits and hares] (1%).

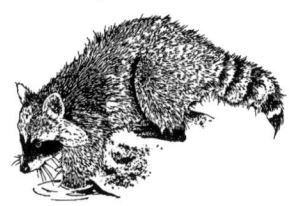

Raccoons are a major rabies reservoir in the east

Outbreaks of rabies infections in these terrestrial mammals are found in broad geographic regions across the United States. Geographic boundaries of currently recognized reservoirs for rabies in terrestrial mammals are shown on the map below based on 2001 data from the CDC.

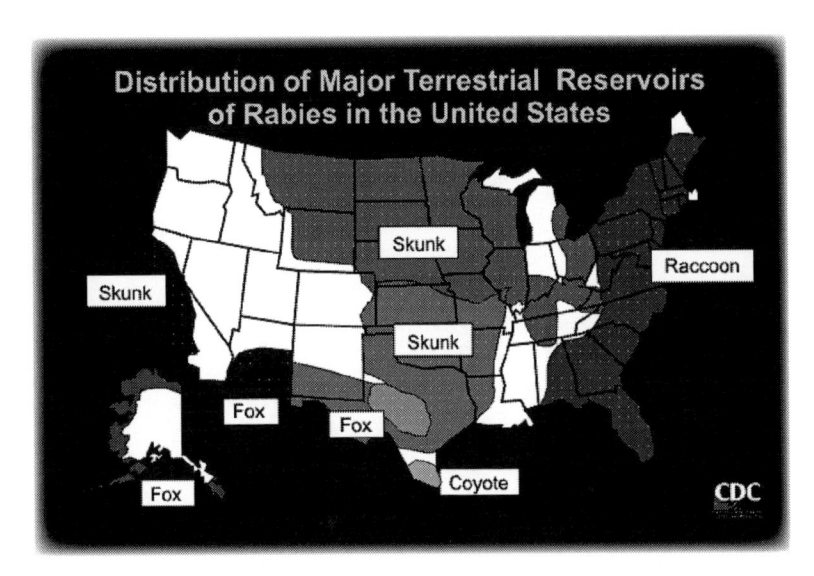

Distribution of Major Terrestrial Reservoirs of Rabies in the United States

In the U.S., bats and raccoons are the animals most often transmitting rabies to humans.

There is a special problem with bat rabies: Between 1990 and 2000, a total of 24 of 32 (75%) of U.S. human rabies cases were caused by bats. In 92% of these cases, however, there was no documentation of a bite. The Centers for Disease Control

(CDC) is now recommending treatment even in the absence of a demonstrable bite or scratch if contact <u>might</u> have occurred. Examples include a sleeping person who awakens to find a bat in the room, or if a bat is found in a room with an unattended child or with a mentally disabled or intoxicated person.

Raccoons have accounted for the largest percentage of animal rabies cases reported to the CDC since 1990. In 2004, 37.5 percent of all rabies cases among animals in the U.S. occurred among raccoons. Raccoon rabies is most common in 20 eastern states but in 2004, 12 of these states actually reported a decrease in the number of rabid raccoons.

First thing to do if you suspect an animal may have rabies is to leave it alone (except see *Capturing Stray Bats Indoors*, below), second thing is to contact the local health department or animal control.

Capturing Stray Bats Indoors

Stray bats often end up in homes in late summer. There may be a roost in the house or they may be young bats simply exploring their territory.

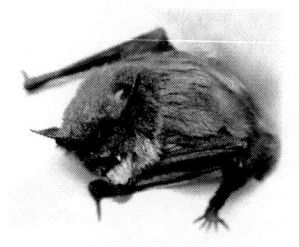

People can be bitten or scratched by a bat and not even know it

photo © Michelle Hamel/iStockphoto

Any time a bat is found in living areas, it should be captured and tested for rabies unless human contact can absolutely be ruled out. People, especially children and the impaired, can be bitten or scratched by a bat and may not be able to tell anyone. Rabies can also be transmitted if a rabid bat's saliva gets into eyes, nose, mouth, or an open wound. You should not release bats captured in a room where there was a sleeping person until you have talked to your local health department to determine whether the bat needs to be killed and tested.

Bites and Scratches

Trapping and otherwise handling live animals poses risk of being bitten and scratched. Here are some safety guidelines:

- Do not try and trap or handle wildlife unless you have training in the proper methods of animal control.
- Be careful with your fingers and other body parts around live traps containing wildlife.
- Wear animal-handling gloves with bite and crush protection suited to the animal.

- Use animal control poles and/or graspers to rescue, restrain, or capture animals.
- Use snake hooks or snake tongs if a snake might be poisonous or if you need to reach inside a void.

> *First Aid for Animal Bites and Scratches*
> - If you are bitten or scratched by an animal, immediately wash the wound with soap and water.
> - Clean the bite by allowing it to bleed and get medical help at once.
> - If bitten or scratched by a loose dog or cat, confine it if you can safely do so. If it's a wild animal, try to capture or kill it without damaging the head.
> - Contact your physician and the local health department.
> - Get a rabies vaccination if the animal is or might be rabid.

Ectoparasites

Birds, rodents, and other wildlife can harbor a wide range of ectoparasites including fleas, ticks, mites, and lice. Some can transmit disease to pets, wildlife, and people (Lyme disease, typhus, and plague). Some wildlife ectoparasites will also infest and feed on people, including technicians trying to control wildlife.

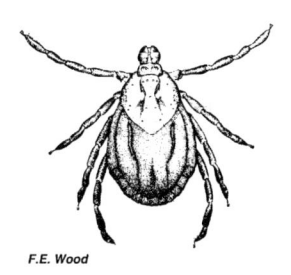

F.E. Wood

The American dog tick will also infest and feed on people

> *Precautions Against Wildlife Ectoparasites*
> - Be alert to the risk of ectoparasites when controlling wildlife.
> - Use repellents when necessary.
> - Wear gloves and long sleeves.
> - In heavy infestations, consider treating the area with an insecticide/acaracide before beginning your control program.

Capturing Nuisance Animals with a Pole or Snare

Even if you do very little nuisance wildlife control, it can be useful to have a catchpole on hand, and know how to use it. Also called a snare pole, this device is basically a long stick with an adjustable noose at one end. The noose, which is made of a loop of cable, is placed over the animal's head and then tightened from the back end of the pole to hold the animal in place.

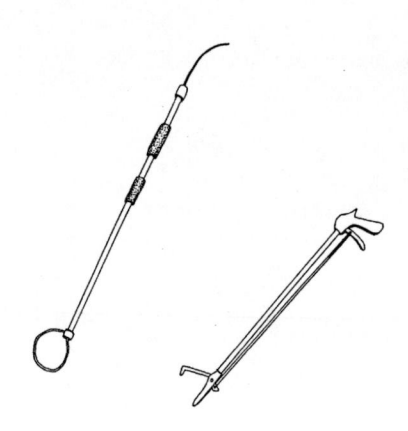

Catchpoles are used by animal control officers and nuisance wildlife control operators to capture and restrain dogs, coyotes, feral cats, foxes, alligators, beavers, bobcats, raccoons, opossums, etc. and snakes until they can be caged. Be sure to wear heavy leather or Kevlar gloves when attempting to capture or restrain an animal.

Commercial catchpoles start at around $20. Some commercial catchpoles swivel so the animal can twist without suffocating. Some lock once the cable is pulled tight but also have a quick-release mechanism. Some catchpoles for small animals have a vice-grip closure at the end of the pole instead of a noose.

You can make your own catchpole from a 3 to 4 foot long hollow metal or PVC tube. Use a length of plastic-coated steel cable (or rope), double it in half and feed it through the tube until a loop comes out one end. Tie off the opposite loose end to keep it from being pulled through the tube. Use the cable at that end to tighten the noose around the animal's neck.

Be very careful in your use of a catchpole. Take care not to strangle or injure the animal. Keep the animal in the noose no longer than absolutely necessary. If a dog's tongue appears blue in color, slacken the noose. Cats can suffocate easily in a head noose; it's better to place the noose over the head and then over one front leg.

Catchpoles for snakes are usually somewhat modified and are called snake sticks, snake hooks, or snake tongs. Snake tongs pin the snake's head to the ground so that it can be safely picked up just behind the head. Don't apply too much pressure or you can injure the snake's spine. Once restrained, pick it up just behind the jaws with your thumb and forefinger and support the rest of its body with your other hand. Place the snake into a garbage can with lid or a cage for transport and relocation. (See also *Snakes* in *Stinging And Venomous Pests*.)

Key Points to Remember—Wildlife

- √ *Do not try to trap or handle wildlife unless you have training in the proper methods of animal control.*
- √ *Be careful with your fingers and other body parts around live traps containing wildlife.*
- √ *Wear animal-handling gloves with bite and crush protection suited to the animal.*
- √ *If you are bitten by an animal, immediately wash the wound with soap and water, allow it to bleed.*
- √ *If bitten or scratched by a wild animal, try to capture or kill it without damaging the head, if it's a pet, try and confine it.*
- √ *Contact your physician and the local health department if you are bitten or scratched.*
- √ *If there's any chance that the animal was rabid, you <u>must</u> get the vaccine.*
- √ *Raccoons and skunks are the most likely animals to be rabid.*
- √ *You can be attacked and infested by certain ectoparasites of wildlife.*
- √ *Catchpoles use a noose to capture and restrain wild animals.*

REVIEW QUESTIONS

The questions that follow relate to the key points under each topic. The answer key follows the questions.

Accident Reporting

1. If an on-the-job incident results in an injury or health impact, the details always should be documented in writing. TRUE or FALSE?

2. List three categories of information that should be included in a written accident report:

   _____

   _____

   _____

3. An accident report should include the names and affiliations of any eyewitnesses. TRUE or FALSE?

Alcohol and Drugs

4. Alcohol and drugs affect your ability to _____, _____, and _____.

5. Name the drug that is most often abused by employees:

6. Over-the-counter and legal prescription drugs may make you an unsafe driver. TRUE or FALSE?

7. If you use an over-the-counter or prescription drug that could affect your performance, you should:

   a) stop using it during work hours

   b) notify your supervisor that you take the drug

   c) take a smaller dosage of the drug

8. If you know that a coworker has a drug problem, you should talk to him or her, or discuss it with a supervisor. TRUE or FALSE?

Allergy

9. An allergic reaction to an insect sting is uncomfortable but is never life-threatening. TRUE or FALSE?

10. If you think you may be having an allergic reaction to an insect sting, you should _____ or _____

11. To reduce your exposure to allergens from insects, mites, and mice when working in a heavily infested account, you should wear a _____, _____, and _____

12. If you are allergic to latex (natural rubber), you should:

    a) tell your supervisor

    b) stop wearing gloves when required during pesticide applications

    c) stop wearing a respirator when required during pesticide applications

13. Repeated exposure to mouse allergens can cause hay fever-like symptoms. TRUE or FALSE?

14. It's okay to use peanut-based baits around children with peanut allergies as long as the children know about the bait. TRUE or FALSE?

Asbestos

15. List three of the many places you might find asbestos:

    _____

    _____

    _____

16. Asbestos fibers that are inhaled can increase the risk of _____

17. Asbestos materials that are undamaged and undisturbed are relatively safe. TRUE or FALSE?

18. If asbestos flooring is undamaged, you can safely drill into it without taking any precautions. TRUE or FALSE?

19. You should not work around crumbling asbestos unless you have been trained in the proper safety procedures. TRUE or FALSE?

20. You should assume that all vinyl floor tiles and sheet flooring contain asbestos if the flooring was installed before:

    a) 1981   b) 1990   c) 1997

21. If you're unsure whether a building material contains asbestos, you should assume that it does and act accordingly. TRUE or FALSE?

Attics and Crawlspaces

22. List three safety precautions to take before entering an attic:

    _____

    _____

    _____

23. List three precautions to take when power-spraying or power-dusting in an attic, crawlspace, or other area with poor ventilation:

    _____

    _____

    _____

24. Besides your own electric tools, what electric shock risk do you face in attics and crawlspaces?

Bird and Bat Roosts

25. Bird and bat droppings are most dangerous:

    a) when they are disturbed

    b) when they are wet or damp

    c) when they become airborne

    d) all of the above

    e) a and c

26. Anyone working in an old bird or bat roost should always assume a potential disease risk. TRUE or FALSE?

27. List the two major diseases you could get from working around accumulated bird or bat droppings:

    _____

    _____

28. After working in a bird or bat roost, if you develop flu-like symptoms that won't go away, you should:

29. What special and additional health concern is associated with bats?

Bloodborne Pathogens

30. List the two major diseases spread by contact with blood, body fluids, or medical waste:

    _____

    _____

31. You could be exposed to bloodborne pathogens if you work in a nursing home. TRUE or FALSE?

32. It's safe to touch medical waste, bandages, blood or bodily fluids as long as you are wearing a respirator. TRUE or FALSE?

33. If your clothing is accidentally contaminated with blood or body fluids, you should remove it, but avoid touching the contaminated area. TRUE or FALSE?

34. If you have to perform CPR (cardiopulmonary resuscitation) on someone, you should use what piece of special safety equipment?

35. If you accidentally splash blood in your eyes, the first thing you should do is:
    a) notify your supervisor
    b) flush your eyes with lots of running water
    c) remove your clothes
    d) put on goggles

Pest Control Technician Safety Manual

Compressed Gas Cylinders

36. The main risk from improper handling of compressed gas cylinders is a condition called hand-arm vibration syndrome. TRUE or FALSE?

37. The Occupational Safety and Health Administration (OSHA) regulates the safe handling of compressed gas cylinders. TRUE or FALSE?

38. List any five guidelines established by the Compressed Gas Association for handling compressed gas cylinders:

   _____

   _____

   _____

   _____

   _____

39. If you find that a fumigant cylinder is leaking, evacuate the area whether you stop the leak or not. TRUE or FALSE?

Confined Spaces

40. OSHA requires a permit before a technician can enter certain confined spaces that are:

   a) especially hazardous

   b) below ground

   c) in public facilities

   d) in industrial sites

   e) none of the above

41. Most technicians have to enter permit-required confined spaces on a regular basis. TRUE or FALSE?

42. Grain storage bins, silos, and hoppers are not usually considered to be permit-required confined spaces. TRUE or FALSE?

43. OSHA exempts sewers from its permit-required confined spaces program. TRUE or FALSE?

44. Before you can enter a sewer, you must:

    a) have permission from the owner of the sewer

    b) have a permit signed by an entry supervisor

    c) follow the confined spaces programs of both your company and the sewer owner.

    d) all of the above

    e) a and c

45. List any three of the many requirements that must be met before you can enter a permit-required confined space:

    _____

    _____

    _____

46. If a coworker has an emergency in a confined space your first priority is to conduct a rescue as quickly as possible. TRUE or FALSE

Driving and Vehicle Safety

47. Seat belts must be used any time your vehicle is in motion. TRUE or FALSE?

48. Describe the "two-second" rule of safe driving:

49. It's safer to park your vehicle so that you can _____ when you leave, rather than having to back up.

50. You should inspect your vehicle once a month to make sure that all systems are operating properly. TRUE or FALSE?

51. You can safely store pesticides in the cab of your vehicle as long as they are in their original containers with original labels intact. TRUE or FALSE?

52. To prevent vehicle rollover, you should carry heavy, bulky items on top of your vehicle whenever possible. TRUE or FALSE?

Pest Control Technician Safety Manual

53. List three items of safety equipment that DOT-regulated commercial vehicles must carry:

   _____

   _____

   _____

54. A buildup of static electricity can start a fire if a gas can is filled while sitting on _____ or _____.

Electric Shock

55. Why should you never remove a grounding prong on an electrical plug?

56. List two types of protection used by tool manufacturers to help protect you from electric shock:

   _____

   _____

57. You should always use a GFI, which is short for _____ _____, when using any electrical tool in a wet area.

58. When working near electrical circuits or other sources of electricity, you should avoid:

   a) using a metal ladder

   b) using water-based pesticides

   c) using a duster that has a metal spout

   d) all of the above

   e) a and c

59. A GFI will protect you from electric shock if you drill into a hidden electrical cable. TRUE or FALSE?

60. If you can't get inside during a thunderstorm, you should take shelter in your vehicle. TRUE or FALSE?

| 220 |

Ergonomics and Musculoskeletal Disorders

61. List three general causes of repetitive stress injury:

    _____

    _____

    _____

62. Hand-arm vibration syndrome sometimes occurs when vibrating hand tools are used for extensive periods. TRUE or FALSE?

63. What are two symptoms of hand-arm vibration syndrome?

    _____

    _____

64. To avoid hand-arm vibration syndrome when using a hammer drill or similar tool, you should schedule a ten-minute break every hour. TRUE or FALSE?

Fiberglass Insulation

65. Fiberglass can harm you only if you inhale the airborne fibers. TRUE or FALSE?

66. The worksite where you are most likely to come in contact with fiberglass insulation is: _____

67. If you must disturb fiberglass insulation, you should:

    a) wear a respirator

    b) wear coveralls, head covering, and goggles

    c) use a fan to circulate the air

    d) all of the above

    e) a and b

Fire

68. Your first concern if a fire is discovered should be putting it out immediately. TRUE or FALSE?

69. If pesticides are burning, you should never attempt to fight the fire. TRUE or FALSE?

70. You should coat the burning surface using a side-to-side motion when using which type of fire extinguisher?

    a) dry chemical fire extinguisher

    b) foam type fire extinguisher

71. You should curve the discharge up slightly so that it falls lightly when using which type of fire extinguisher?

    a) dry chemical fire extinguisher

    b) foam type fire extinguisher

72. When using a flammable product around a gas stove, you should first:

Firearms

73. List any three safety practices when handling a firearm:

    _____

    _____

    _____

74. You should keep firearms loaded and locked in a case when not in use. TRUE or FALSE?

75. A benefit of airguns is that they are not powerful enough to cause serious injury or property damage. TRUE or FALSE?

First Aid

76. When giving first aid to a victim, you should:

    a) wear gloves

    b) avoid contact with blood

    c) use a mouth mask when performing CPR

    d) all of the above

    e) a and b

77. According to guidelines from the American Heart Association, if an adult is unconscious, you should first administer CPR (cardiopulmonary resuscitation), then call an ambulance. TRUE or FALSE?

Flashlights

78. Flashlights can explode due to a buildup of hydrogen gas in the battery compartment. TRUE or FALSE?

79. It can be hazardous to open a flashlight near an open flame. TRUE or FALSE?

Hand and Power Tools

80. List two things to check before using a cutting hand tool:

    _____

    _____

81. List any three of the many precautions to follow when using electric power tools:

    _____

    _____

    _____

82. To use a grounded tool in an ungrounded receptacle, first remove the third prong on the plug. TRUE or FALSE?

83. After a jack has been used to lift a load, what must you do before working underneath?

84. Lasers used for bird dispersal can damage a person's eyes if aimed incorrectly. TRUE or FALSE?

Head Injury

85. OSHA requires that you wear a protective helmet to protect yourself from what two different hazards?

    _____

    _____

Pest Control Technician Safety Manual

86. All approved protective helmets will protect you against these two different hazards. TRUE or FALSE?

87. Why shouldn't you wear a helmet with leather straps or a leather sweatband when applying pesticides?

Heat and Cold

88. List two of the three personal health factors that can increase your risk of heat illness:

    _____

    _____

89. Mental confusion, inability to sweat, hot, dry skin and fever are characteristics of what life-threatening condition?

90. Which of the following are first aid procedures to treat heat illness?
    a) lie down in a cool place, feet raised and clothing loosened
    b) avoid drinking any fluids
    c) splash or sponge water on face, neck, and arms
    d) all of the above
    e) b and c
    f) a and c

91. Cold weather injuries occur most often when the air temperature is between 35 and 40 degrees F. TRUE or FALSE?

92. The symptoms of pesticide poisoning and the symptoms of either heat stress or hypothermia can be very similar. TRUE or FALSE?

Hookworm or "Creeping Eruption"

93. If you have inflamed, itchy tracks on your skin you should:

94. You can be infected with hookworm by contact with the feces of:
    a) raccoons   b) dogs   c) cats
    d) all of the above e) a and c

95. Hookworm infestation causes numbness and blanching of the skin. TRUE or FALSE?

96. List two ways to protect yourself from hookworm when working in a crawlspace:
    _____
    _____

Hospitals and Other Medical Facilities

97. Hospital staff is trained to notify you in advance of any biohazards you may face in the facility. TRUE or FALSE?

98. You should check in with the person in charge at each location that you service. TRUE or FALSE?

99. Give two requirements that you must meet before working in medical areas posted as hazardous:
    _____
    _____

Ladders

100. List two acceptable ladders to use if you are going to be working around electrical wires or electrical equipment:
    _____
    _____

101. How far away from a building should the base of a non-self-supporting 20 foot ladder be placed?
    a) 1/2 of its length   b) 1/4 of its length
    c) one foot   d) two feet

102. If you are using a ladder to get on a roof, it should extend at least _____ feet above the roof.

Pest Control Technician Safety Manual

103. Which of the rungs of an extension ladder are unsafe to stand on?

104. What must you do before transporting a ladder on a vehicle?

Lifting and Back Safety

105. The number one rule regarding lifting is to:

106. If you're not sure if you can lift a load, you should make sure you bend from the waist to lift it safely. TRUE or FALSE?

107. You should never lift a heavy load higher than:

108. You should make sure you have a cleared place to set a load down before you start to lift it. TRUE or FALSE?

Lockout/Tagout

109. Lockout prevents a person from turning on a piece of equipment by locking or bolting the disconnect switch. TRUE or FALSE?

110. Explain what tagout is:

111. Pest control technicians are subject to OSHA's lockout/tagout rules if they work around a piece of equipment that could:

112. After you have serviced a piece of tagged equipment, you should remove the tag to show that it is ready for use. TRUE or FALSE?

Molds

113. Only "toxic molds" cause health effects in humans. TRUE or FALSE?

114. Molds can grow on grains and stored foods, as well as on building materials. TRUE or FALSE?

115. What is the one most important thing that molds require for growth?

   a) carbon dioxide

   b) moisture

   c) sunlight

   d) air flow

116. The greatest risk to technicians working around molds is inhaling air-borne mold spores. TRUE or FALSE?

Natural Gas

117. A hissing sound can be an indication of a natural gas leak. TRUE or FALSE?

118. If you're inside a building and you smell a strong gas odor, you should:

   a) use the customer's phone to call for emergency help

   b) turn off all lights

   c) alert others and leave the building

   d) all of the above

Needlesticks

119. If you are stuck by a used needle, the first thing you should do is:

   a) write an incident report

   b) notify your supervisor

   c) wash and disinfect the wound

120. You could end up with hepatitis if you accidentally stick yourself with a used needle. TRUE or FALSE?

121. You should never reach into areas you can't see like under a bed or in a trash can unless you have a first aid kit nearby. TRUE or FALSE?

Pest Control Technician Safety Manual

Noise

122. Exposure to loud noises, such as using a hammer drill, can cause hearing loss. TRUE or FALSE?

123. When noise exceeds safe levels, ear plugs, cotton balls, or ear muffs can be used for hearing protection. TRUE or FALSE?

124. Approved hearing protection will prevent hearing loss or injury no matter how loud the noise. TRUE or FALSE?

125. Reusable ear plugs should be cleaned and disinfected regularly. TRUE or FALSE?

Pesticides and Other Chemicals

126. Your customer is at greater risk of exposure to pesticides than you are. TRUE or FALSE?

127. OSHA's Hazard Communication Standard:

    a) is a monthly safety newsletter

    b) requires that employees be given information to protect themselves from hazardous chemicals

    c) specifies which government agencies should be notified in case of a pesticide spill

    d) is a set of guidelines for chemical manufacturers

128. An MSDS, which stands for _____ _____, is a guide to the potential hazards of a pesticide or other hazardous chemical.

129. A pesticide with a WARNING signal word on its label is considered to be:

    a) slightly toxic   b) moderately toxic

    c) highly toxic   d) nontoxic

130. The main risk to a technician using a dust formulation is inhalation hazard. TRUE or FALSE?

131. Skin absorption of pesticide is generally faster with which one of these pesticide formulations?

   a) bait
   b) dust
   c) wettable powder
   d) emulsifiable concentrate

132. Besides being flammable, gasoline can injure you or make you sick by what three routes?

   _____
   _____
   _____

Pesticide Poisoning

133. When spraying, a technician usually faces the greatest risk of pesticide exposure through inhalation. TRUE or FALSE?

134. The genital area absorbs pesticide more rapidly than surrounding areas of the body. TRUE or FALSE?

135. Many pyrethroid insecticides can cause a skin reaction in sensitive individuals; describe it:

136. List four ways you could have oral exposure to a pesticide:

   _____
   _____
   _____
   _____

137. If you're applying pesticides in a poorly-ventilated, restricted space like an attic, your greatest poisoning risk is from:

   a) dermal exposure
   b) oral exposure
   c) inhalation exposure
   d) eye exposure

138. If you splash pesticide in your eye, you must wash it out for at least 15 minutes. TRUE or FALSE?

Pest Control Technician Safety Manual

Pesticide PPE

139. When must you wear a respirator?

140. List two <u>medical</u> conditions that can make someone unable to use a respirator safely :

    _____

    _____

141. You should check the condition and the seal of your respirator once a week. TRUE or FALSE?

142. The newer 100-series HE respirator filters:

    a) replace the older HEPA filters

    b) are purple in color

    c) protect against viruses, bacteria, allergens, and asbestos

    d) all of the above

143. A leather glove is considered to be "chemical-resistant" if you are applying only pesticide granules. TRUE or FALSE?

144. Where should you store your respirator?

145. Prescription eyeglasses qualify as protective eyewear. TRUE or FALSE?

146. If you take your work clothes home to be washed, how can you protect your family from exposure to any pesticide residues in the clothing?

Pets and Guard Dogs

147. You should never enter an account with a dog present and no one home, unless you are sure that the dog poses no threat. TRUE or FALSE?

148. If you service commercial accounts, you should:

    a) periodically ask about guard dogs

    b) not enter dog-guarded areas after hours unless you have the customer's assurance that the dog won't bite

    c) carry dog treats

    d) all of the above

149. If bitten by a dog, you should wash out the bite, see a physician, and be sure to get a copy of the animal's rabies vaccination. TRUE or FALSE?

Poison Ivy

150. Each poison ivy leaf is made up of _____ distinct leaflets.

151. Long sleeves, long pants, and gloves will help protect you when working around poison ivy. TRUE or FALSE?

152. If you've been exposed to poison ivy, you should follow which procedure?

    a) clean the area with rubbing alcohol, wash it with cool water, then shower using soap

    b) wash the area with soap and water and then apply rubbing alcohol

    c) wash the area thoroughly with plain hot water, no soap

    d) don't wash the area, apply calamine lotion

153. You should wash your clothes separately from other laundry, and clean shoes and tools as soon as possible after exposure to poison ivy. TRUE or FALSE?

154. Burning poison ivy is the only way to remove it without fear of an allergic reaction. TRUE or FALSE?

Power-Dusting and Power-Spraying

155. When should you inspect power dusters or power-spraying equipment?

156. You should wear a respirator when operating gasoline-powered spray equipment in enclosed or unventilated areas. TRUE or FALSE?

Pest Control Technician Safety Manual

157. List two ways to avoid walking through your application when using a power duster or power sprayer:

    _____

    _____

158. To avoid airborne residues, drift, and splashback when power-spraying, you should:

    a) use a high application pressure

    b) use a low application pressure

    c) use a nozzle that produces smaller droplets

    d) none of the above

    e) b and c

159. Before opening the tank of a compressed air power duster, you should release the air pressure. TRUE or FALSE?

Radiation

160. Exposure to excessive radiation may cause mutations in your unborn children. TRUE or FALSE?

161. The hazard warning sign for radiation is a magenta or black triangle on a red background. TRUE or FALSE?

162. You should never enter a radiation area without:

    _____ and _____

Rodents

163. Which of these is a health risk from handling rodents?

    a) bites   b) scratches

    c) fleas and ticks   d) diseases

    e) all of the above

164. If you are handling live rodents, you should wear disposable plastic gloves. TRUE or FALSE?

| 232 |

165. Rodent carcasses should be disposed of in a:

166. Which of the following is NOT true about hantavirus?
    a) it is spread through the urine, saliva, or feces of a mouse
    b) the house mouse is the most common carrier of the disease
    c) it is usually spread by inhalation in dusty areas
    d) it is most common in the western United States

167. In hantavirus areas, you should wear a dust mask when cleaning up or disturbing large accumulations of rodent droppings. TRUE or FALSE?

168. A rare bacterial disease caused by a bite or scratch from a rodent is:
    a) rabies   b) hookworm
    c) malaria   d) ratbite fever

169. The "Black Death," or _____, is a rare disease that can be spread by the bite of an infected flea or by handling an infected animal.

170. Lymphocytic Choriomeningitis (LCM) is a virus that can be spread to humans by contact with house mouse droppings, urine, saliva, or nest material. TRUE or FALSE?

171. When cleaning up rodent-infested sites, it's important to use a disinfectant on surfaces, dead rodents, rodent nests, and on your gloves before removing them. TRUE or FALSE?

Roofs

172. You should be trained in fall protection before you work on a roof where there is a risk that you could fall _____ feet.

173. A fall protection system is a device that will keep you from falling more than 20 feet before being caught. TRUE or FALSE?

174. What should you do before putting on a body harness?

175. List two types of acceptable fall protection systems:

   _____

   _____

176. You do not need to have a fall protection system in place if:

   a) the work is of short duration and limited exposure

   b) you are working on a ladder

   c) installing the fall protection system is just as hazardous as doing the job itself

   d) any of the above

   e) a and c

177. List two electric shock hazards to avoid when working on roofs:

   _____

   _____

Scaffolds

178. Scaffolds and their supports must be capable of supporting their load with a twofold safety factor. TRUE or FALSE?

179. Planking used in scaffolding:

   a) must be scaffold-grade planking

   b) must extend over end supports no less than 6 inches

   c) must overlap a minimum of 12 inches or be secured

   d) all of the above

Slips, Trips, and Falls

180. To help avoid slips, trips, or falls, you should:

   a) use a flashlight when working in low light areas

   b) clean up spills immediately

   c) wear shoes with smooth leather soles

   d) all of the above

   e) a and b

181. Older workers are no more likely to slip or fall, and no more likely to be injured, than younger workers. TRUE or FALSE?

Spills

182. A large pesticide spill or leak should be handled by a specially trained and equipped emergency crew. TRUE or FALSE?

183. The three "C's" to remember in a spill emergency are:

   _____

   _____

   _____

184. Before you get near a spill, you should:

185. If a spill is moving towards a body of water, you should immediately block or redirect it. TRUE or FALSE?

186. Your state requires that you report any spill over _____ (list specific amount, if applicable):

187. You should report a pesticide spill to your office before you take any action to control it. TRUE or FALSE?

188. A quick way to contain a leak from a liquid pesticide container is to:

Stinging and Venomous Pests

189. When controlling wasps or bees, you should:
   a) use a flashlight to locate the opening of the nest
   b) make noise to frighten the guard wasps or bees
   c) use extra precautions if you are using a ladder
   d) all of the above
   e) a and c

Pest Control Technician Safety Manual

190. What pesticide product can protect you when inspecting for bees or wasps?

191. Why must you remove a honey bee's stinger quickly from your skin?

192. To protect yourself when inspecting for fire ants under rocks, put your hands under the rocks and flip them over quickly. TRUE or FALSE?

193. Before reaching into a hidden or dark area in scorpion country, you should:

194. A scorpion can grab on and sting you more than once. TRUE or FALSE?

195. The bite of the black widow spider has no immediate painful effect but can leave a slow-healing ulcerated wound. TRUE or FALSE?

196. If attacked by Africanized bees you should cover your head with a shirt or cloth and run for shelter. TRUE or FALSE?

197. If bitten by a poisonous snake, you should:

    a) apply ice   b) apply a tourniquet

    c) get medical help   d) suck out the venom

198. What two items of protective equipment should you be wearing if you are trying to capture a poisonous snake?

    _____

    _____

Stress

199. List three possible problems from long-term job stress:

    _____

    _____

    _____

200. Stress is a mental condition that does not affect you physically. TRUE or FALSE?

201. Physically fit people find it easier to manage stress. TRUE or FALSE?

202. _____ between management and employees can help resolve stressful situations.

Tetanus

203. Tetanus, or lockjaw, is a disease transmitted by the bite of an infected flea. TRUE or FALSE?

204. You should get a booster tetanus shot:

   a) every year   b) every other year

   c) every 5 years   d) every 10 years

205. If you are 50 years old or older, you should automatically check with your physician about the status of your tetanus vaccination. TRUE or FALSE?

Tick-transmitted Diseases

206. List the three most common tick-transmitted diseases:

   _____

   _____

   _____

207. Blacklegged ticks are most common in treeless, grassy areas. TRUE or FALSE?

208. A skin rash can be one of the symptoms for which three tick-transmitted diseases?

   _____

   _____

   _____

209. List three safety precautions to take if you work in a tick-infested area:

   _____

   _____

   _____

Pest Control Technician Safety Manual

Tuberculosis (TB)

210. Tuberculosis (TB) is transmitted from an infected person through airborne particles which can be spread by normal air circulation. TRUE or FALSE?

211. If an area is posted as a tuberculosis area, do not enter unless you have (list two):

   _____

   _____

Vaccinations

212. Under what two circumstances should a technician consider getting vaccinated for hepatitis B?

   _____

   _____

213. A flu shot provides protection for about:

   a) 3 months

   b) 1 year

   c) 3 years

   d) life

214. There is no preventative vaccine for rabies. TRUE or FALSE?

Violence

215. What is the best way to avoid road rage?

216. List three common situations that pose risk of violence on the job for a pest control technician:

   _____

   _____

   _____

217. List three ways to reduce the risk of violence when servicing an apartment complex:

   _____
   _____
   _____

218. What is the best way to defuse a confrontation between you and another person?

Warehouses

219. When working in warehouses, you must use the personal protective equipment specified by the warehouse. TRUE or FALSE?

220. "Dock jumping" means jumping from a loading dock to the ground, rather than using the stairs. TRUE or FALSE?

221. When doing rodent control in a warehouse, you are at risk from:

   a) forklift and pallet jack traffic

   b) shifting of stacked product

   c) chemical exposure

   d) all of the above

   e) a and b

Warning Signs

Briefly describe what the illustrated warning signs mean to you on the job.

222.

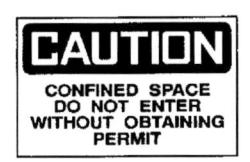

CAUTION
CONFINED SPACE
DO NOT ENTER
WITHOUT OBTAINING
PERMIT

Pest Control Technician Safety Manual

223.

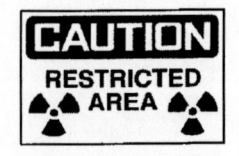

CAUTION
RESTRICTED AREA

224.

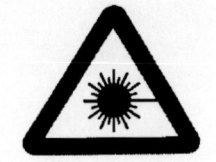

225.

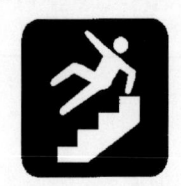

226.

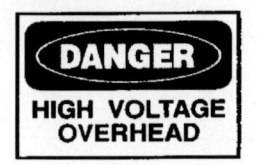

DANGER
HIGH VOLTAGE OVERHEAD

227.

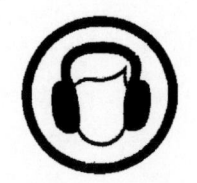

228.

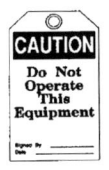

229.

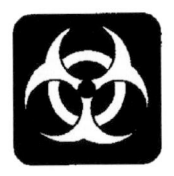

230.

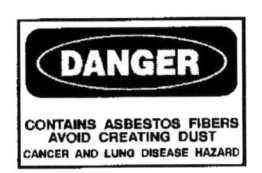

231.

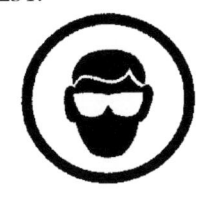

232.

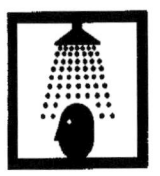

233.

> THIS EQUIPMENT CONTAINS PCB Polychlorinated Biphenyls CAPACITOR(S)

Wildlife

234. What is the purpose of animal-handling gloves?

235. If bitten by a wild animal, you should:
    a) use a compress to stop the bleeding
    b) wash the wound and let it bleed
    c) apply a tourniquet
    d) apply meat tenderizer

236. You should never attempt to capture a wild animal that has bitten you. TRUE or FALSE?

237. To protect your hands when trapping or handling wildlife, you should:
    a) make sure you've been trained in animal control safety procedures
    b) avoid putting your fingers near live traps containing wildlife
    c) wear animal-handling gloves
    d) all of the above

238. If you are bitten, you must wait for symptoms to see if you need to get rabies shots, even if there is only a very small chance the animal was rabid. TRUE or FALSE?

239. Which two animals are most likely to be rabid in the U.S.?

　_____

　_____

240. If a wild animal is acting unusually friendly and tame, you should suspect rabies. TRUE or FALSE?

241. You can get rabies from a bat even if you haven't been bitten. TRUE or FALSE?

242. Catchpoles are noose devices that are designed to choke and kill wild animals. TRUE or FALSE?

243. Give three types of ectoparasites that can be found on wild animals and that can bite people or pets:

    _____

    _____

    _____

ANSWERS TO REVIEW QUESTIONS

1. TRUE
2. background information; description of accident; outcome
3. TRUE
4. think; move; react
5. alcohol
6. TRUE
7. b
8. TRUE
9. FALSE
10. get to a physician (or) call 911
11. respirator, goggles, long sleeves
12. a
13. TRUE
14. FALSE
15. any three of the places listed on page 13
16. cancer, especially lung cancer
17. TRUE
18. FALSE
19. TRUE
20. a
21. TRUE
22. any three of the following: assess the hazards; take action to protect yourself; wear appropriate PPE; carry a good flashlight; make sure the attic ladder is safe
23. any three of the precautions listed on page 19
24. loose or dangling electric lines or cables
25. e
26. TRUE
27. histoplasmosis; cryptococcosis
28. see a physician

29. rabies
30. human immunodeficiency virus (HIV); hepatitis B virus
31. TRUE
32. FALSE
33. TRUE
34. mouth mask
35. b
36. FALSE
37. TRUE
38. any five of the guidelines listed on page 27
39. TRUE
40. a
41. FALSE
42. FALSE
43. FALSE
44. d
45. any three of the following: must be authorized; must be trained; written program in place; permit system in place; air testing/monitoring in place; safety equipment on hand; attendants on hand; planned rescue program
46. FALSE
47. TRUE
48. a visual and counting system using a roadside landmark that helps you gauge your following distance from the vehicle in front of you as you count 1001, 1002
49. pull forward
50. FALSE
51. FALSE
52. FALSE
53. Any three of the following: fire extinguisher, spare fuses for brake lights, emergency flares or emergency triangles, retroreflective tape:
54. plastic truck bed liner (or) in the trunk
55. you could get a serious or fatal electric shock

Pest Control Technician Safety Manual

56. any two of the following: grounding prongs on plugs; double-insulated tools; ground fault interrupters (GFIs)
57. ground fault interrupter
58. d
59. FALSE
60. TRUE
61. any three of the following: repeating the same motion; working in an awkward position; using a lot of force; repeatedly lifting heavy objects; using hand or power tools; working in the cold
62. TRUE
63. any two of the following: tingling; numbness; pain; blanching
64. TRUE
65. FALSE
66. an attic
67. e
68. FALSE
69. TRUE
70. a
71. b
72. make sure the stove is off and temporarily turn off the pilot light
73. any three of the precautions listed on pages 68-69
74. FALSE
75. FALSE
76. d
77. FALSE
78. TRUE
79. TRUE
80. sharpness; condition
81. any three of the precautions listed on pages 77-78 (or even 75-76)
82. FALSE
83. block the jack with a jack stand or other support
84. TRUE

85. injury to the head; electrical shock
86. FALSE
87. leather can absorb pesticides
88. any two of the following: overweight; diabetes; certain medications
89. heat stroke
90. f
91. FALSE
92. TRUE
93. see a physician
94. d
95. FALSE
96. wear coveralls and gloves (no bare skin); wash up afterwards
97. FALSE
98. TRUE
99. any two of the following: proper authorization; proper training; protective equipment if necessary
100. wooden ladder; fiberglass ladder
101. b
102. three
103. the top three rungs
104. make sure it's securely attached
105. think before you lift
106. FALSE
107. your waist
108. TRUE
109. TRUE
110. placing a special warning tag on the disconnect switch or valve of a piece of equipment to warn others against using it

111. cause injury by starting up or releasing energy

112. FALSE

113. FALSE

114. TRUE

115. b

116. TRUE

117. TRUE

118. c

119. c

120. TRUE

121. FALSE

122. TRUE

123. FALSE

124. FALSE

125. TRUE

126. FALSE

127. b

128. material safety data sheet

129. b

130. TRUE

131. d

132. breathing vapors; swallowing it; spilling on skin

133. FALSE

134. TRUE

135. tingling or burning and numbness

136. any four of the following: smoking or chewing tobacco with contaminated hands; biting contaminated fingernails; eating with contaminated hands; drinking with contaminated hands; blowing on a hose or nozzle; accidentally splashing it in mouth; swallowing it directly; wiping mouth with contaminated hand or sleeve; accidentally applying it to objects that then go into mouth

137. c

138. TRUE

139. whenever inhaling airborne contaminants can affect your health

140. any two of the following: heart trouble; lung trouble; use of certain medications

141. FALSE

142. d

143. FALSE

144. in an airtight container (protected from dust, chemicals, and the elements)

145. FALSE

146. store and wash them separately from family laundry

147. TRUE

148. a

149. TRUE

150. three

151. TRUE

152. a

153. TRUE

154. FALSE

155. before each use

156. FALSE—NEVER operate a gasoline engine in an enclosed or unventilated space

157. apply pesticide to the side; walk backwards away from the direction of application

Pest Control Technician Safety Manual

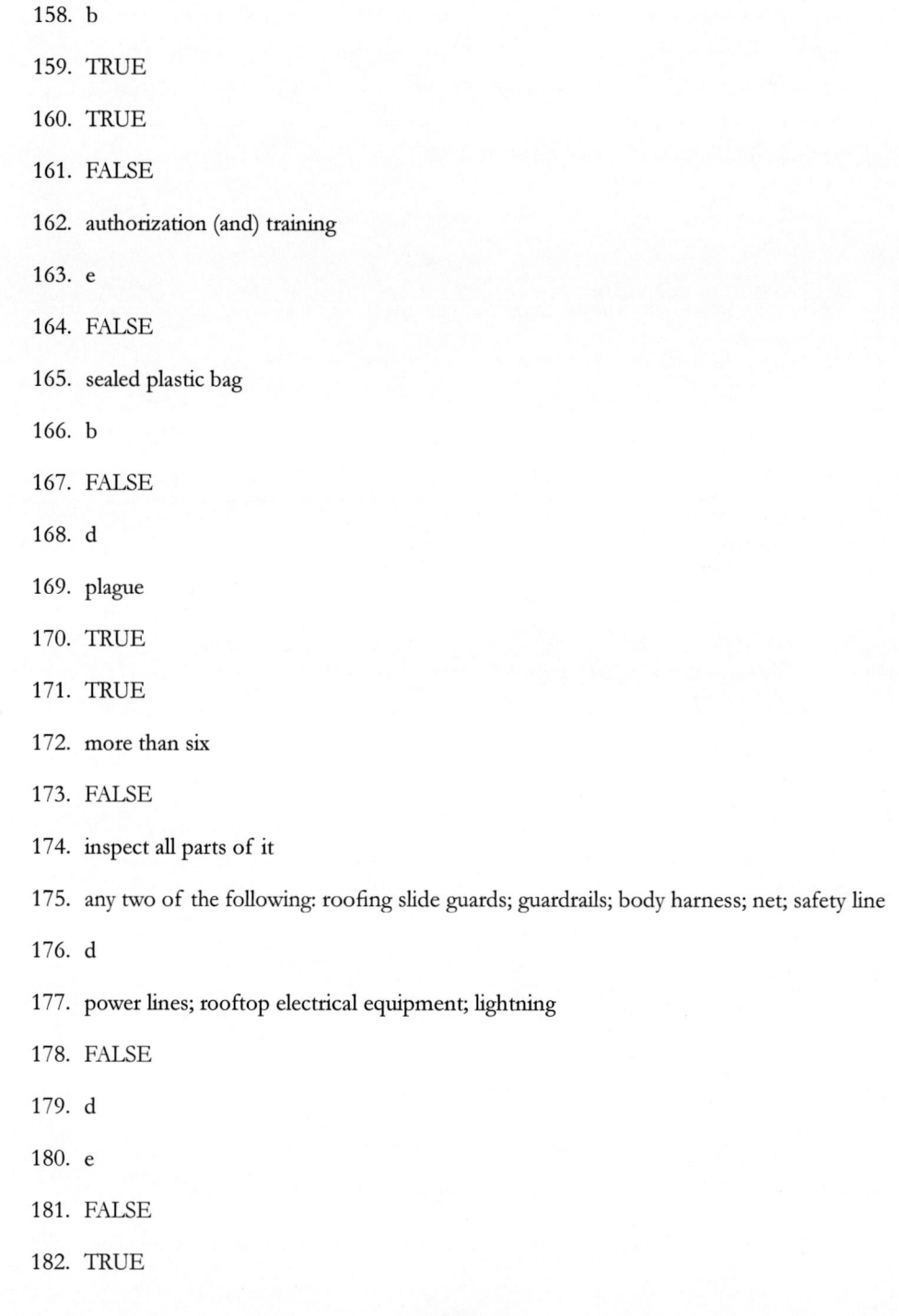

158. b

159. TRUE

160. TRUE

161. FALSE

162. authorization (and) training

163. e

164. FALSE

165. sealed plastic bag

166. b

167. FALSE

168. d

169. plague

170. TRUE

171. TRUE

172. more than six

173. FALSE

174. inspect all parts of it

175. any two of the following: roofing slide guards; guardrails; body harness; net; safety line

176. d

177. power lines; rooftop electrical equipment; lightning

178. FALSE

179. d

180. e

181. FALSE

182. TRUE

183. control; contain; clean up

184. put on the appropriate PPE

185. TRUE

186. varies by state and often by pesticide—just be sure you know your state's regulations

187. FALSE

188. place it in a plastic bucket

189. c

190. a quick-freeze wasp spray

191. it continues to pump out venom

192. FALSE

193. put on gloves

194. TRUE

195. FALSE

196. TRUE

197. c

198. leather boots, and leather or animal-handling gloves

199. any three of the following: cardiovascular disease; back problems; neck problems; depression; burnout; unsafe work practices; headaches; sleep disturbances; difficulty concentrating; short temper; upset stomach; job dissatisfaction; low morale

200. FALSE

201. TRUE

202. discussions (communication)

203. FALSE

204. d

205. TRUE

206. Lyme disease; Rocky Mountain spotted fever; ehrlichiosis

207. FALSE

208. Lyme disease; Rocky Mountain spotted fever; ehrlichiosis

209. any three of the precautions listed on pages 192-193

210. TRUE

211. proper authorization; proper respirator; respirator training

212. if he/she regularly works in hospitals or other medical facilities; if he/she is trained and authorized to provide emergency first aid

213. b

214. FALSE

215. drive gently

216. any three of the situations listed on page 199

217. any three of the precautions listed on page 200

218. be willing to back down

219. TRUE

220. TRUE

221. d

222. warns of a "permit-required confined space"; there are a long list of requirements you must meet before you may enter it

223. there is a radiation hazard and you shouldn't enter without authorization and training

224. there could be a laser operating in the area

225. there is a slip and fall hazard

226. there is high voltage overhead; you should take care when using ladders, bee poles, or when treating overhead

227. you should wear hearing protection

228. there is a tagout program in place and you should not operate this equipment

229. there are biohazards in the area

230. there is a dangerous asbestos risk; do not enter without proper training, authorization, and personal protective equipment

231. you must wear eye protection

232. there is an emergency shower nearby

233. there could be a PCB hazard, and you should take precautions to avoid exposure

234. to protect against bites and scratches from live animals

235. b

236. FALSE

237. d

238. FALSE

239. raccoons; skunks

240. TRUE

241. TRUE

242. FALSE

243. fleas; ticks; lice; mites